Supercharge
Your Diet

By Sam Rice and available from Headline

The Midlife Method:
How to lose weight and feel great after 40

Supercharge Your Diet

Ten Easy Ways to Get Everything You Need
from Your Food

SAM RICE

Copyright © Sam Rice 2022

The right of Sam Rice to be identified as the author of
the work has been asserted by her in accordance with the
Copyright, Designs and Patents Act 1988.

First published in 2022 by HEADLINE HOME an imprint of
HEADLINE PUBLISHING GROUP

1

Apart from any use permitted under UK copyright law, this publication may only be reproduced, stored, or transmitted, in any form, or by any means, with prior permission in writing of the publishers or, in the case of reprographic production, in accordance with the terms of licences issued by the Copyright Licensing Agency.

Every effort has been made to fulfil requirements with regard to reproducing copyright material. The author and publisher will be glad to rectify any omissions at the earliest opportunity.

Cataloguing in Publication Data is available from the British Library

Trade paperback ISBN 978 1 4722 9795 2
eISBN 978 1 4722 9794 5

Illustrations by Caitlin Rose

Publishing Director: Lindsey Evans
Senior Editor: Kate Miles
Copy editor: Tara O'Sullivan
Proofreader: Margaret Gilbey
Indexer: Ruth Ellis

Designed and typeset by EM&EN
Printed and bound in Great Britain by Clays Ltd, Elcograf S.p.A.

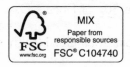

MIX
Paper from
responsible sources
FSC® C104740
www.fsc.org

Headline's policy is to use papers that are natural, renewable and recyclable products and made from wood grown in well-managed forests and other controlled sources. The logging and manufacturing processes are expected to conform to the environmental regulations of the country of origin.

HEADLINE PUBLISHING GROUP
An Hachette UK Company
Carmelite House
50 Victoria Embankment
London EC4Y 0DZ

www.headline.co.uk
www.hachette.co.uk

Contents

The Recipes 109

About Me

My journey to becoming a food and health writer began in 2012 following the death of my youngest brother Ben from type 1 diabetes, an incurable autoimmune condition. Slowly, the disease took its toll on his body, his microbiome was ravaged, and his weight plummeted as his body struggled to get adequate nutrition from the food he was eating.

The shock of losing Ben taught me that health is a privilege and my own issues were self-inflicted: too many empty calories from processed foods; not enough fruit and vegetables to deliver the nutrients my body needed; too much alcohol and too little respect for my gut health, despite having had digestive issues for years.

As the cliché goes, I woke up one morning and decided enough was enough. I spent the next few years experimenting in the kitchen, trying to find healthy foods I loved to eat, and I quickly learned the power of the food we eat to heal and sustain. I also lost weight – not because I was dieting, but because I was eating the right balance of foods in the right amounts, so my digestive system could work efficiently.

My first book, *The Midlife Kitchen*, was the culmination of everything I learned in those years. Co-written with award-winning author and journalist Mimi Spencer, it went on to be a *Sunday Times* bestseller. My most recent book, *The Midlife Method: How to lose weight and feel great after 40*, has also helped many thousands of midlifers build a better relationship with food.

Apart from books, I write freelance for many publications, notably the *Daily Telegraph*, with a focus on making good nutrition accessible to all. I am a member of the Guild of Food Writers and a graduate of Leith's Nutrition in Culinary Practice course, which is the best training of its kind in the UK, with a focus on translating nutritional theory into delicious food.

But that's enough about me; it's time to supercharge your diet.

Introduction

Eating healthily is easy, right? Just make sure you have your five-a-day (or is it eight now?); eat plenty of fibre (hmmm, what exactly is fibre, and how much do I need?); cut down on meat (but which types of meat, and by how much?); eat more fish (but is that sustainable, and is farmed fish OK?); ensure you are getting all the necessary vitamins and minerals; oh, and don't forget prebiotics and probiotics for gut health. Maybe it's not so easy, after all . . .

The confusing and often misleading information available from both official sources and social media has created a nutritional minefield. You'd be forgiven for taking the ostrich approach and sticking your head in the sand, which was certainly how I felt ten years ago, before I decided to get to grips with my own nutrition.

But unfortunately, our poor-quality Western diets are known to be the cause of many chronic illnesses,[1] and simply ignoring the issue is not something we can afford to do if we want to stay fit and healthy into our later years. The latest figures from the UK Health Security Agency speak for themselves:[2]

- Only 29% of adults are eating the recommended five portions of fruit and vegetables a day.

- The average fibre intake in adults is 19g per day, well below the recommended 30g per day.

- Ultra-processed foods account for 56.8% of total energy intake in the typical UK diet; the ideal figure would be close to zero.

- Currently, 30,000 deaths a year are linked to obesity, and the cost to the NHS is estimated at £500 million a year.[3]

But there is some good news. A new study from researchers in Norway has found that adopting a healthier diet can extend lifespan by six to seven years in middle-aged adults, and could increase lifespan in young adults by about ten years.[4] The recommendations included:

- eating more legumes (beans, peas and lentils)

- increasing intake of wholegrains

- eating nuts on a regular basis

- consuming less red and processed meat

These are useful rules of thumb for a healthier diet and a longer life, but how can we put this into practice? How can we really be sure we are getting everything we need from our food? That's where this book comes in. With a little knowledge and a well-stocked larder, you don't need to be a dietitian to supercharge your diet. Let's get started.

What Exactly *Do* We Need From Our Food?

Understanding this question is at the heart of this book, and it's not as complex as you might think. Essentially, food is made up of macronutrients (carbohydrates, fat and protein) and micronutrients (vitamins and minerals). The *Oxford English Dictionary* definitions of these terms are as follows:

> **Macronutrient:** A type of food (e.g. fat, protein, carbohydrate) required in large amounts in the diet.

> **Micronutrient:** A chemical element or substance required in trace amounts for the normal growth and development of living organisms.

But already there's a complication. What is a 'large' amount and what is a 'trace' amount? How do we know we are getting the right quantities of macro- and micronutrients from our food? Most countries provide nutritional guidelines; indeed, the UK government's latest recommendations, published in 2016, are shown overleaf.[5]

If those tables of figures mean absolutely nothing to you, you are not alone. In fact, as our understanding of good nutrition evolves, these kinds of blanket recommendations are being discredited. Professor Tim Spector, author of the bestselling book *Spoon-Fed: Why Almost Everything We've Been Told About Food is Wrong* is not a fan:

> We are used to listening to government advice and guidelines about nutrition, health and wellness. But can the same health advice really apply to a population of millions of individual humans with their own lifestyles and unique physiology? Is the one-size-fits-all an appropriate base for healthcare policy?[6]

He makes an excellent point; indeed, personalised nutrition is gathering pace as the next big thing in health. At the moment, it's relatively difficult and expensive to access, so until we are all

Supercharge Your Diet

Government recommendations for energy, salt, dietary fibre, macronutrients, vitamins and minerals for males and females aged 19+ years

Age (years)	19–64		65–74		75+	
Gender	Males	Females	Males	Females	Males	Females
Energy(MJ/day)	10.5	8.4	9.8	8.0	9.6	7.7
Energy (kcal/day)	2500	2000	2342	1912	2294	1840
Salt (g/day) [less than]	6.0	6.0	6.0	6.0	6.0	6.0
Dietary fibre (g/day)	30	30	30	30	30	30
Macronutrients						
Protein (g/day)	55.5	45.0	53.3	46.5	53.3	46.5
Fat (g/day) [less than]	97	78	91	74	89	72
Saturated fat (g/day) [less than]	31	24	29	23	28	23
Polyunsaturated fat (g/day)	18	14	17	14	17	13
Monounsaturated fat (g/day)	36	29	34	28	33	27
Carbohydrate (g/day) [at least]	333	267	312	255	306	245
Free sugars (g/day) [less than]	33	27	31	26	31	25
Vitamins						
Vitamin A (µg/day)	700	600	700	600	700	600
Thiamin (mg/day)	1.0	0.8	0.9	0.8	0.9	0.7
Riboflavin (mg/day)	1.3	1.1	1.3	1.1	1.3	1.1
Niacin equivalent (mg/day)	16.5	13.2	15.5	12.6	15.1	12.1
Vitamin B6 (mg/day)	1.4	1.2	1.4	1.2	1.4	1.2
Vitamin B12 (µg/day)	1.5	1.5	1.5	1.5	1.5	1.5
Folate (µg/day)	200	200	200	200	200	200
Vitamin C (mg/day)	40	40	40	40	40	40
Vitamin D (µg/day)	10	10	10	10	10	10
Minerals						
Iron (mg/d)	8.7	14.8/8.7*	8.7	8.7	8.7	8.7
Calcium (mg/day)	700	700	700	700	700	700
Magnesium (mg/day)	300	270	300	270	300	270
Potassium (mg/day)	3500	3500	3500	3500	3500	3500
Zinc (mg/day)	9.5	7.0	9.5	7.0	9.5	7.0
Copper (mg/day)	1.2	1.2	1.2	1.2	1.2	1.2
Iodine (µg/day)	140	140	140	140	140	140
Selenium (µg/day)	75	60	75	60	75	60
Phosphorus (mg/day)	550	550	550	550	550	550
Chloride (mg/day)	2500	2500	2500	2500	2500	2500
Sodium (g/day)	2.4	2.4	2.4	2.4	2.4	2.4

* 19–50y / 50–64y

able to tap into precise information about how our bodies metabolise the food we eat, we are stuck with these general guidelines.

So where does that leave us in trying to ensure we get what we need from our food? Knowing which kinds of foods deliver all the macro- and micronutrients we need for optimal health will help, as will ensuring that, *overall*, our diets are balanced and based on nutritional principles we know to be true, like having plenty of fibre, eating a good range of plant foods and minimising sugar and heavily processed foods.

This book will empower you to do this by explaining these basic nutritional principles and helping you translate them into daily practice in the kitchen. But first, we need to understand how our nutritional requirements change over time.

Our Changing Nutritional Requirements Over Time

Healthy eating is important at any stage of life and, broadly speaking, what's good for you at 20 is also good for you at 70, but our nutritional needs do vary somewhat as we age. It's useful, then, to understand these changes so you can shift where your focus is food-wise according to your body's needs.

Childhood and teens

Growing bodies need plenty of calories, but unfortunately these all too often come in the form of ultra-processed foods (UPFs). Ensuring children and teens get as many of their calories as possible from whole foods is the best way to make sure they are getting the nutrition they require. As they get older, you have less control over what they eat outside the home, but as long as what they are getting at home is balanced and healthy, they should still be getting adequate nutrition.

Macronutrients

Complex carbohydrates are the best source of energy for your growing child, such as wholegrain bread and wholemeal pasta, brown rice, potatoes (preferably in their skins), oats and other wholegrains. These foods should form around 50% of what's on their plate.

Additionally, each meal needs to contain some lean protein for growth, maintenance and repair of the body in the form of lean meat, fish, dairy, eggs, pulses, beans and soya products, such as edamame, miso and tofu, if you can persuade them to eat it.

Fat is an essential part of your child or teen's diet. It plays a key role in brain development, forms the building blocks of hormones, and helps the body absorb the fat-soluble vitamins A, D, E and K. But it needs to be the right type of fat and in the right amounts.

Aim to have oily fish once a week (salmon, mackerel or even sardines on toast), use plenty of olive oil and encourage them to eat nuts and seeds in various forms. Including these in smoothies is a good trick, and nut butters are also an easy win (try making your own omega-3 version, see page 151). You could also make healthy oat, nut and seed snack bars like the Oaty Fruit Slices on page 236.

Micronutrients

While we often focus on children's physical health when it comes to nutrition, there's a growing emphasis on the role nutrition plays in the mental health of our younger population. A 2021 study by the University of East Anglia found that the consumption of at least five portions of fruit and vegetables a day had a positive correlation with mental well-being in teenagers.[7]

The best policy when it comes to feeding kids and teens is to keep it simple; find the fruit and veg they like and have them in plentiful supply at home. Berries are often called nature's vitamin pills, and are almost universally enjoyed; buy frozen ones out of season. As mentioned above, smoothies are an excellent way to load up on healthy ingredients, so get them to experiment with their favourite fruit and veg combos. There are some delicious and nutritious smoothie recipes to try later in the book.

Other considerations for kids when it comes to micronutrients are calcium for bone growth, along with vitamin D, which helps the body to absorb it. Calcium is found in dairy and soy products, leafy green vegetables and fish that contain edible bones (sardines on toast again!). The best way to get vitamin D is from sunshine on the skin, so kick them outside when the weather is nice. There are some food sources of vitamin D, such as oily fish, eggs and mushrooms, so having those on the menu will also help.

All kids, but particularly teenage girls whose periods have begun, will benefit from a good supply of iron from lean meat, liver (although this could be a hard sell!), wholegrain cereals, pulses, beans, nuts, sesame seeds, leafy dark green vegetables and dried fruit, especially apricots. Remember that vitamin C is required for iron absorption; the best sources are citrus fruits, berries, peppers, tomatoes, broccoli and potatoes. A good tip is to have a bowl of satsumas on the kitchen table so they can grab one as a quick snack when they pass through.

In our twenties and thirties

The aim in these two decades of life is to develop good eating habits and to lay the foundations for future health. It can be easy in early adulthood to feel invincible; our bodies can take a lot of punishment with seemingly few consequences. But you might just be storing up problems for the future.

Macronutrients

Rather than worrying too much about the proportions of the three macronutrients you are eating, it's better, at this stage of life, to focus on the quality of the carbs, protein and fat in your diet. If you head for the ready-meal section at the local supermarket when food shopping, the likelihood is that the quality won't be great. Cooking simple food at home using whole foods should be the goal.

If you enjoy exercise and have an active lifestyle, you'll need plenty of energy from complex carbs, and perhaps now is the time to be more adventurous. Experiment with new foods, like having quinoa rather than rice and sweet potatoes rather than regular ones. Eating a variety of plant foods will pave the way for good gut health in the future.

It's easier to build muscles and strong connective tissue when we are younger, and by doing the groundwork early we can minimise problems in later life such as sarcopenia or age-related loss of muscle mass. Also, consider the quality of the protein you are eating; move away from processed food and red meat, and favour leaner cuts. Eggs, dairy and plant proteins should also feature regularly in your diet.

In your twenties, your brain is still developing, and it's a good time to start thinking about your heart health to reduce the risk of high blood pressure and coronary disease in the future. One of the best ways to do this is to eat brain- and heart-friendly fats from oily fish, avocados, nuts, seeds and olive oil. Love it or hate it, the millennials' favourite, avocado toast, has probably done wonders for their future heart health.

Micronutrients

A 2018 study by the UK National Diet and Nutrition Survey (NDNS)[8] found that a large number of adults in their twenties and thirties were failing to achieve the minimum recommended intakes for 12 key nutrients: vitamins A, C, B2 and B12, plus folate (B9), calcium, iron, magnesium, potassium, zinc, selenium and iodine.

It seems, then, that this age group would do well to focus on their micronutrient intake generally. The best way to do this is to eat plenty of colourful fruits and vegetables. The popular phrase 'eat the rainbow' should be the mantra in early adulthood. For more specific information on food sources for the key micronutrients, see pages 84–5.

Midlife

Midlife, broadly the years from age 40 to 60, is characterised by hormonal changes that can lead to a redistribution of fat, which tends to accumulate around the middle. This is especially true in menopausal women, as the decline in oestrogen levels seen during this time may promote belly-fat storage.

Men will also tend to increase their levels of visceral fat, the fat stored deep inside the belly around the organs, which is a risk factor for cardiovascular disease. If you are a man in this age category and have developed the tell-tale D-shaped belly, it's time to act to avoid future health problems.

Macronutrients

A subtle shift in macro balance can be helpful in midlife. When we are younger, 50–60% of our calories should come from carbohydrates; in midlife, that can reduce to around 45%, with more coming from protein and fat. The extra protein will support muscle mass, which begins to decline from around the age of 30 unless active steps are taken to prevent this. Healthy fats are important to protect heart and brain health. Choose monounsaturated fats from healthy sources like olive oil.

But a word of caution. While reducing carbs a little may be beneficial, don't be tempted to cut them out completely. Very low-carb diets, like keto, have been popular in recent years as a means to rapid weight loss, and, indeed, for certain medical reasons, a low-carb diet may be appropriate, for example if you are pre-diabetic. But special circumstances aside, complex carbohydrates play an important role in endocrine (hormone) balance, as well as sustaining energy levels, and should feature in your daily diet. Focus on wholegrains, as they also contain that all-important fibre, critical for gut health as well as appetite regulation.

Micronutrients

In midlife, our focus shifts to extending our healthspan – that is, the number of fit and active years we have ahead. Working against us is oxidative damage to our cells caused by free radicals. These may sound like cool dudes, but they are in fact the cause of many non-communicable diseases, such as cancer and type 2 diabetes, as well as chronic inflammation.

Introduction

Eating plenty of polyphenols, also called antioxidants, which are found in the pigments of brightly coloured fruits and vegetables, as well as in dark chocolate and red wine in moderation (hurrah!), is the best way to see off those pesky intruders.

Midlife can also be a very stressful time of life. A study by Penn State University found that people aged 45 to 65 feel more stressed now than their counterparts did in the 1990s as they deal with the challenges of kids, work, ageing parents and the constant pull to stay connected.[9]

The key nutrient when it comes to dealing with stress and anxiety is magnesium. It helps the body relax and can help you sleep better, which is critical when it comes to managing stress. Magnesium is found in lots of whole foods, including pumpkin seeds, almonds, leafy greens, bananas, avocados and fish. If you eat a varied and well-balanced diet, there's no reason why you should be deficient in magnesium, but it's definitely worth keeping a particular eye on in midlife.

And one for the ladies: if you are heading towards the menopause, then give your hormones a helping hand by keeping your phytoestrogens topped up. Soy beans (enjoy as edamame, tempeh and tofu) and flaxseeds (which you can grind and put into smoothies, porridge and overnight oats) are good sources, and you should also eat lots of broccoli and other cruciferous veg (sprouts, cabbage, cauliflower, kale), which contain indole-3-carbinol, a plant chemical known to increase oestrogen metabolism.

Later life

Once we are over 60, the real fun and games begin. A general reduction in physical activity and a lower BMR (basal metabolic rate) caused by a decrease in muscle mass means that our caloric need is less. What this means in practice is that we need to get all our nutrition from fewer calories. Quite a challenge.

The physiological changes we experience as we get older can also compound the problem. Our guts become less efficient as we age, and this affects nutrient absorption. Older people may also experience a loss of appetite due to hormonal changes and impairment of the senses of smell, taste and vision, which all contribute to the enjoyment of food.

Macronutrients

Sarcopenia, or loss of muscle mass, really starts to kick in from the age of 65. Keeping physically active is absolutely key to minimising its effects, and from the perspective of diet, upping your protein intake is the single best line of defence. One study followed 2,066 elderly people over three years.[10] It found those who ate the most protein daily lost 40% less muscle mass than people who ate the least over a three-year period. That's a pretty compelling statistic.

The problem is that many older people are not eating enough. Another study found that 35% of participants were not eating adequate protein to maintain muscle mass and function; it recommended that for optimal muscle synthesis, people over 65 should aim for a protein intake of 25g, three times a day.[11]

The best concentrated sources of protein are meat, fish, eggs and dairy. To give you some idea of what 25g of protein looks like, it would be around 100g chicken or steak, 125g fish, four eggs, 250g Greek yogurt, 100g Cheddar, 230g cottage cheese or 250g lentils. Lots of recipes in this book have 25g or more of protein, so look out for those later on if you need to up your intake.

Healthy fats and complex carbs are still important in the diet as we get older. Eat plenty of wholegrains, nuts, seeds, olive oil and seafood – all key features of the Mediterranean diet, which is still recognised as the best overall diet for longevity.

Micronutrients

I mentioned earlier a decrease in our energy needs as we get older, which means we have less food from which to gain nourishment.

Introduction

This problem can be compounded by a reduction in stomach acid associated with ageing, which leads to poor absorption of vitamins and minerals. This condition is known as atrophic gastritis, and studies have estimated that it affects 20% of the elderly population.[12]

To counter this, it's even more important to eat nutrient-dense foods. Focus on leafy greens, oily fish and shellfish, brightly coloured fruit and vegetables, eggs, wholegrains, nuts and seeds. Yes, it's a familiar roll call, but for good reason: these are some of the most nutritious foods on the planet.

Two micronutrients that deserve special mention for seniors are calcium and vitamin D. As discussed above, calcium helps build and maintain healthy bones to reduce the risk of fractures, while vitamin D helps the body absorb calcium.

Unfortunately, studies have found that the gut tends to absorb less calcium with age, which is largely due to vitamin D deficiency, since ageing can make the body less efficient at producing it.[13] In addition, older people may find it more difficult to spend time outside for sun exposure due to mobility issues, and as we age our skin becomes thinner, reducing its ability to make vitamin D.

Getting as much of these critical nutrients as possible from the diet is important, but this is one scenario where it may be advisable to take a good-quality supplement. And on the subject of supplements . . .

Can't I Just Take Supplements?

If the heaving shelves of our chemists and health-food shops are anything to go by, we are a nation of supplement guzzlers. It's estimated that almost 20 million people in the UK take some form of daily food supplement,[14] and the global dietary supplements market was valued at a whopping £115 billion in 2021.[15]

Now this book is about getting everything you need nutritionally from your food, so in that sense it is anti-supplement, because I truly believe that if we know how to nourish ourselves properly, we can largely ditch the pills. A 2018 survey looking at consumer attitudes and behaviour in relation to food supplements for the Foods Standards Agency found that most people take supplements through sheer force of habit, and that they do not know if they are actually making any difference.[16] Because such products were viewed as being fairly benign, it was better to be safe than sorry.

So, is there any problem with that? Well, I think there is. First of all, our bodies are designed to eat food, nature's packages of macro- and micronutrients that are broken down into their constituent parts by our digestive processes and used as required. Our guts are not designed to digest the concentrated formulations found in supplements, and there is little evidence of how much benefit they provide.

In fact, a 2020 study looking at the health effects of vitamin and mineral supplements published in the *British Medical Journal* found no evidence that supplements protect against non-communicable diseases such as cardiovascular disease, cancer or type 2 diabetes.[17] They also found that an adequate intake of nutrients from foods, but not supplements, was associated with a lower risk of all-cause mortality. More evidence that the best way to nourish ourselves is by eating well, not popping pills.

Introduction

It may interest you to know that supplements in the UK are subject only to the laws governing food; in other words, as long as they are safe to ingest, they can be sold. Unlike medicines, there is no compulsory testing or requirement to prove efficacy of the product. When it comes to supplements, it is very much a case of buyer beware – and let's not forget they can also be very expensive.

Some supplementary considerations

Why are you taking supplements?

Take a look at pages 84–5 for the main food sources of the various vitamins and minerals. If you are eating these things on a regular basis, you are probably not deficient and so do not need to supplement.

Have you looked at the ingredients list of your supplements?

You might be surprised at the long list of things that go into those little pills and capsules. Do you know what they all are? There may well be ingredients that, while not necessarily harmful, are not things you particularly want to ingest. One supplement I looked at contained beef gelatine, glycerol (as a humectant), titanium dioxide (for colour), palm oil (probably not sustainably sourced) and emulsifiers.

Have you considered the contraindications of taking supplements?

There's a tendency to think that by taking supplements, all you are doing is filling in the nutritional cracks; in other words, it's all upside. But this isn't always the case and it's important to take your own medical history into account when deciding whether to take supplements. For example, if you have a personal or family history of cancer, it's best to avoid vitamin A/beta-carotene supplements, as clinical studies have shown that taking more than the recommended dosage increases cancer risk. It's this kind of information that you generally won't find plastered on the front of supplement packets, so you need to do your homework.

It IS possible to take too much

Overloading on vitamins and minerals can be harmful, and if you take a lot of supplements without checking exactly what's in them, and the doses of each component, you may be doing more harm than good. For example, too much vitamin C or zinc can cause nausea, diarrhoea and stomach cramps. Too much selenium can lead to hair loss, gastrointestinal upset, fatigue, and mild nerve damage.[18] More is not necessarily more when it comes to supplements.

I'm hoping this book will convince you that for most of us, supplements aren't necessary, and your money is better spent on good-quality, natural whole foods. However, if you decide you still want to take them, then aim to do so in a targeted and informed way.

Having said all that, there may still be times when supplements are advisable. This book is written for omnivores who don't have any specific medical conditions; in other words, it assumes you can eat all types of foods and your body will be able to digest and process those foods adequately.

If you are on a restricted diet for personal, ethical or medical reasons, then targeted supplementation may be required, and there are some other specific scenarios where it is recommended. For example, vegan and vegetarian diets can be lacking in B12, iron, zinc and omega-3. In the winter months, when sunshine is in scarce supply, vitamin D supplements are useful for most people, and there are also certain supplements recommended during pregnancy. There may also be a case for those who struggle to eat a balanced diet, for example children who are picky eaters, to take a good-quality multivitamin.

In summary, supplements do have a role to play, but our first line of defence should be what we put in our mouths. With a little knowledge and effort in the kitchen, we can get everything we need from our food. The rest of this book will explain how.

Ten Easy Ways to Get Everything You Need from Your Food

The purpose of this book is to translate your body's nutritional requirements into what you eat and drink every day. I have broken it down into ten simple categories, so that by the end, you'll know what your body needs and why, and how to eat to tick all those nutritional boxes. Some of this will already be familiar to you, and some of it will be new, but none of it is rocket science. Eating well is perfectly possible once you understand the basics.

These are the ten easy ways to get everything you need from your food:

ONE: Switch to complex carbohydrates

TWO: Focus on lean and plant proteins

THREE: Include healthy fats

FOUR: Have 30g of fibre a day

FIVE: Support your gut health

SIX: Get your five-a-day

SEVEN: Get your vitamins and minerals in

EIGHT: Keep an eye on calories

NINE: Snack smart

TEN: Think about what you drink

We will explore each of these categories in detail over the following pages. I've also created 80 recipes designed to deliver optimal nutrition, so you can be sure you are putting your newfound knowledge into practice. Let's start with carbs.

ONE

Switch to Complex Carbohydrates

What are carbohydrates, and why does my body need them?

Carbohydrates are organic compounds found in plants that, when eaten and digested by the body, are converted into glucose (a form of sugar), which the body then uses for energy. The glucose circulates in the blood to power the muscles, nervous system and brain. When there's too much glucose in the blood, the hormone insulin is released by the pancreas, and it's converted into glycogen to be stored in the muscles and liver, or into fat for storage in the fat cells.

Carbohydrates exist in three forms in our food: sugar, starch and fibre.

> **Sugar** – These are short-chain or 'simple' carbohydrates, such as glucose, fructose and sucrose, which are quickly absorbed into the blood stream.

> **Starch** – These are longer 'complex' chains of sugar molecules, which take longer to be broken down into glucose by the digestive system.

> **Fibre** – Fibre is a type of carbohydrate our bodies cannot digest, but it is crucial for gut health and proper functioning of the bowels.

Is sugar really 'toxic'?

One of the more confusing food narratives of recent years has centred around the 'toxic' nature of sugar, often in the context of it having caused the obesity crisis and the rocketing rates of type 2 diabetes. In truth, the body is well designed to metabolise glucose as an energy source. In fact, it's an important macronutrient, and carbohydrates, mainly in the form of fruit and vegetables, also deliver other important micronutrients.

When it comes to sugar and health, there's really only one distinction you need to make, and that's between the 'intrinsic' sugars that occur naturally in foods, for example the fructose found in fruit and vegetables and the lactose in milk, and 'added' or 'free' sugars, refined sugars that usually come in liquid or granulated form.

Eating too much 'free' sugar, for example in sugary drinks, snacks and processed foods, can cause problems because it is easily absorbed by the body, causing blood sugar spikes that, over time, can lead to insulin resistance and potentially to type 2 diabetes.

Although products like honey, maple syrup, coconut sugar and agave syrup are often marketed as 'natural', they aren't chemically all that different to regular white sugar and are still considered free sugars. If you think about it, even bog-standard granulated sugar is extracted from plants (sugar cane or sugar beet), so in that sense, it too is natural.

But surely, I hear you cry, honey and maple syrup contain other nutrients that make them healthier than normal sugar? Again, this is a triumph of marketing over fact. Honey does contain some vitamins and minerals, but they are contained in such small amounts that you'd have to be eating a huge quantity of honey to get them in anywhere near significant enough levels to be beneficial, and at that point, the negative effects of the sugar consumption far outweigh the miniscule nutritional value.

Are sugar substitutes OK?

Sugar substitutes are another nutritional hot potato – no carb pun intended! Studies have shown that replacing sugary foods or drinks with artificially sweetened ones may reduce calorie intake and aid weight loss,[19] and can help those with diabetes to reduce their sugar intake. Conversely, there's some evidence that artificial sweeteners might increase appetite and promote weight gain.[20] Go figure.

It's important to make the distinction between artificial sweeteners, which are effectively chemicals used to sweeten foods (aspartame, acesulfame K, saccharin and sucralose), and plant-based sugar substitutes (stevia, monkfruit sweetener, and sugar alcohols like xylitol and erythritol).

Artificial sweeteners have been linked to various adverse health outcomes, including an increased risk of cancer and metabolic syndrome, but again the evidence is not conclusive. Studies have also indicated that they can upset the balance of the gut bacteria in some people.[21]

Plant-based sugar substitutes may be a better bet, the most common being stevia, which has been shown to lower high blood pressure in people with hypertension[22] and is a helpful sugar alternative for people with diabetes.[23] But, as with chemical sweeteners, stevia can negatively affect the gut microbiome.[24]

Research continues, but to be on the safe side, you may wish to avoid sugar substitutes. Certainly they are not going to confer any great benefit, and in that sense they bring little to the nutritional party.

What are 'good' carbs and 'bad' carbs?

No doubt you'll have heard carbs being described as 'good' or 'bad' in the media, which has had the unhelpful effect of attaching a moral value to certain foods. If you eat that slice of pizza, you're bad, but have a green smoothie and you can pop that health halo back on.

But let's be clear: foods simply exist on a scale of less nutritious to more nutritious; there's no need to label them good or bad, and we certainly shouldn't feel guilty for eating a slice of pizza from time to time! In health terms, we just need to ensure that most of what we eat comes from the more nutritious end of the scale, otherwise it becomes difficult to get what we need from our food.

In the case of carbohydrates, we can divide them into *simple carbohydrates* (the less nutritious ones), such as white bread, fizzy drinks, juices and those processed foods with lots of added sugar, and *complex carbohydrates* (the more nutritious ones), found in wholegrains, vegetables and legumes like peas, beans and lentils.

Aren't low-carb diets healthier?

Whether you call it Atkins, Dukan, keto or paleo, the huge popularity of a low-carb diet with the promise of rapid weight loss means low-carb has been top of the diet pops for decades. The central idea is that by cutting carbs (and therefore glucose) as an energy source, the body will convert fat into molecules called ketones, which can then be used for energy instead. These diets advocate the drastic cutting of carbs and replacing them with protein and fat; in fact, these diets are often high in saturated fat.

There is some good evidence to support the use of low-carb diets in certain circumstances, particularly for people who may be pre-diabetic and need to lose weight, because 'low-carbing', as it has been termed, minimises insulin release. There have also been claims that low-carb diets can help ward off other diseases like cancer and dementia; however, there is currently scant evidence for this.

But the main question mark over low-carb diets has been around heart health. As ketogenic diets are often high in saturated fat, they have the potential to raise blood cholesterol levels, in particular the harmful LDL type of cholesterol, which has been linked to heart disease. Evidence is, again, inconclusive. A 2019 report on the prevention of heart disease by the American Heart Association said low-carb diets were linked with higher death rates,[25] while another study found participants' overall risk score for heart disease fell by 12% after a year on a ketogenic diet.[26]

While the scientists continue to battle it out, the best current advice is to aim for a balanced diet that contains some complex carbs to provide slow-release energy, and plenty of fibre for a healthy gut.

Where do GI and GL come into it?

GI (glycaemic index) and GL (glycaemic load) are terms that have been hijacked by the diet industry as another faddy way to sell weight-loss programmes. In essence, they are simply ways to describe how quickly a particular food raises our blood sugar levels.

GI refers to how quickly the carbohydrates in a food are digested and absorbed; in other words, a low-GI food takes longer to enter the bloodstream and so raises blood sugar levels at a slower pace than a high-GI food.

GL is also concerned with the rate at which a food affects blood sugar levels, but it is more useful in the sense that it also takes into account the portion size. A food may have a high GI, but if it is eaten in a small amount, then it won't have a huge impact on blood sugar levels.

Whether we are talking about GI or GL, our aim nutritionally is to minimise blood sugar spikes, which, as mentioned, are known to increase insulin resistance, a risk factor for type 2 diabetes. Complex carbohydrates are the healthier 'slow-release' type, and as such they are the ones we want to focus on in our diets.

What are the best sources of complex carbs and how much should I eat?

The current guidelines for adults in the UK recommend that half our energy requirements come from carbohydrates. While this is a useful rule of thumb, there are other factors to take into account, such as age and lifestyle.

When we are younger and have a higher energy requirement, as much as 65% of our caloric intake may come from carbohydrates. As we get older, reducing the amount of carbs in favour of protein and fat can be beneficial for the reasons previously discussed.

Lifestyle factors also play a part. Having a physical job or doing lots of exercise will increase your energy requirement, and there are other specific scenarios when you may need to up your energy intake, such as after an operation or illness, or when pregnant.

Switching to eating more complex carbs and minimising simple carbs is one of the best things we can do nutritionally, because our Western diets tend to be so skewed in favour of the latter. Aim to eat more from this first list, and less from the second:

Healthy sources of complex carbohydrates

Fruits and vegetables – Most people don't realise that fruit and vegetables, apart from water, are mainly carbohydrates. They are also excellent sources of many different micronutrients and fibre. A wide range of fruit and vegetables should form the basis of every meal.
  Portion size – For more information on portion sizes for fruit and veg, see the five-a-day section.

Wholegrains – Wholegrains, such as wholegrain bread (ideally freshly baked, not packet sliced) and wholemeal pasta, oats, quinoa, bulgur wheat and brown rice, contain starch and fibre. They are not just a key energy source, but are important for gut health too.
  Portion size – One slice of wholegrain bread or 100g of cooked grains like oats, rice or pasta.

Nuts and seeds – Nuts and seeds are the starting blocks for the next generation of plants, so it makes sense that they are bursting with nutrients. The benefits are too many to mention, but suffice to say they should be eaten on a regular basis.

    Portion size – 30g nuts, 1 tablespoon seeds.

Legumes – Peas, beans, chickpeas and lentils are not just good sources of complex carbs, they are also packed with plant protein and are an excellent, fibre-rich way to keep you feeling full. As such, they can really help with appetite regulation.

    Portion size – 80g or 3 heaped tablespoons of cooked legumes.

Tubers – Sweet potatoes and regular potatoes (eaten with their skin) are not just a good source of starchy carbs; they also contain a surprising amount of micronutrients. Sweet potatoes have beta-carotene in their orange pigment, which is converted into vitamin A, and potatoes are a good source of vitamin C.

    Portion size – Clench your fist: this is your portion size for tubers.

Simple carbohydrates that should be minimised

Soft drinks and juices – Often high in free sugars that will lead to blood sugar spikes.

Most shop-bought breakfast cereals – These are highly refined products, often with lots of added sugar.

Refined grains, including white rice and regular pasta – These products have had most of their fibre removed, and are not as nutritionally dense as their wholegrain equivalents.

Ultra-processed bread and bread products – Your regular sliced bread, bagels, etc. contain lots of additives to extend their shelf-life.

Processed snack foods – All those packet snacks, including cakes, cereal bars, biscuits and crisps, usually contain lots of added sugar as well as unhealthy fats and salt.

Free sugars you have at home – Even the sweeteners we have at home in granulated and liquid form (regular sugar, brown sugar, honey, maple syrup, coconut sugar) should be used judiciously. You are in control of how much you use; a spoonful of honey on your porridge is fine, but if you are a keen baker, you'll be using a lot.

Carbs recap

- Complex carbohydrates are an important source of energy and fibre.

- Intrinsic sugars found in fruit and milk are fine, but limit your intake of added or 'free' sugars.

- Sugar substitutes have been found to negatively affect gut health and do not convey any nutritional benefits.

- Rather than referring to 'good' or 'bad' carbs, just know that some are better for us nutritionally than others.

- Complex carbs are low GI/GL, which keep blood sugar levels stable.

- Approximately half our calories should come from complex carbohydrates (this does vary from person to person).

- The most nutritious sources of carbs are fruit, vegetables, wholegrains (and wholegrain bread and wholemeal pasta), nuts, seeds, peas, beans, lentils, and potatoes (sweet and regular in skins).

Ten easy ways to switch to complex carbs

1. **Eat lots of leaves.** Remember leafy green vegetables are a source of complex carbs and are extremely nutrient-dense. Choose from spinach, chard, kale, pak choy, rocket or watercress. Wilt down to have with your morning eggs, add to a smoothie, make into a lunchtime salad or have as a side dish at dinner.

2. **Don't drink your fruit.** Eat fruit whole rather than drinking juice to make sure you are getting all the lovely fibre. Smoothies are better in that the fibre is largely retained, and you can add grains, nuts and seeds for a better balance – see the Wake-up Smoothie on page 124.

3. **Make fruit your go-to sweet fix.** When you get a craving for something sweet, opt for a piece of fruit. Although fruit contains fructose, or fruit sugar, this is combined with fibre and other micronutrients that won't spike blood sugar in the same way as free sugar.

4. **Only buy wholegrain versions of staple foods.** Some simple swaps to make to your shopping trolley include buying wholegrain, freshly baked bread, wholegrain crackers, wholemeal pasta and brown rice.

5. **Pop in a pouch.** Buy pre-cooked pouches of wholegrains to put in salads and to have as side dishes. They can be quickly heated up in the microwave and spices and herbs added for flavour. Try the Zingy, Grainy, Grated Salad on page 196.

6. **Aim to eat some nuts and seeds daily.** These can be added to porridge, overnight oats or smoothies, or you could try the Wholegrain Granola on page 122.

7. **Chuck in a tin.** Legumes are most convenient when bought in tins. Just drain, rinse and chuck them in. Add lentils to a Bolognese (or a shakshouka – see page 164), beans to a soup or salad and chickpeas to a curry.

8. **Keep the skins on.** When having potatoes, keep the skins on, as this is where the fibre and micronutrients are found. Baked is best, or try making oven-baked wedges tossed in olive oil, salt and pepper, and roasted until crispy.

9. **Roast your roots.** Roasting robust vegetables like sweet potatoes and other root vegetables is easy and delicious. Try making the Roasted Roots with Feta and Mint on page 128. You can always roast more vegetables than you need and blend them with vegetable stock to make a tasty soup.

10. **Sweeten with dates.** Dates are a fibre-rich, whole food, and are just about the healthiest way to add sweetness to whatever you're making. Add to smoothies or chop into porridge, have as a snack or make your own date purée to use in place of other sweeteners by blending with water and a drop of lemon juice.

TWO

Focus on Lean and Plant Proteins

What is protein and why does my body need it ?

Carbohydrates have hogged the health headlines in recent years, but protein is now having its moment in the sun as we realise the crucial role it plays in maintaining healthy bones and organs, in enzyme and hormone production, and in keeping our immune systems functioning optimally. Protein is also a key factor in weight management, as it increases satiety (how full we feel after eating), so we consume less overall, thus making it easier to keep our weight under control.

Another important function of protein is in building and retaining lean muscle. As discussed earlier, muscle mass reduces as we age, which can eventually lead to physical deterioration and reduced mobility. To continue living a full and active life, we need plenty of protein in our diets. It's relevant here to note that protein isn't stored in the body like carbohydrates and fat are, so if we don't get enough from our diets, we will begin to lose muscle.

And now for the science bit. Proteins are long chains of compounds called amino acids. There are 20 different amino acids that are important for health, 11 of which the body can make itself and are referred to as 'non-essential'. The remaining nine are called the 'essential' amino acids; the body cannot make these, and so they have to come from our diets.

Complete proteins contain all nine essential amino acids, and are generally found in animal-based sources such as meat, fish and dairy. Plant-based proteins are mostly *incomplete*, which means that in order to get all the amino acids we require, we need to eat a wide variety of these foods. This is especially important for vegans and vegetarians, whose access to complete proteins is limited. Plant-based proteins include soy foods, legumes, grains and seeds.

What has protein got to do with working out?

You might have seen those buff Insta-influencers clutching their post-workout bowls of 'proats' (a contraction of 'protein oats', or porridge in old money!). Indeed, a whole protein cult has grown up around working out, which can seem rather baffling if your idea of exercise is a brisk walk round the block.

The reasoning behind eating protein after a workout is that exercise, and especially strength training, creates little tears in the muscles, which is why you can feel sore after strenuous exercise. Given protein plays a key role in maintaining and repairing muscles, the theory is that by giving your body a protein boost, it will help the muscle to recover and build.

While this all sounds very plausible, protein deficiency is rare in a Western diet. In fact, the average daily intakes of protein in the UK exceed the RNI (Reference Nutrient Intake) level set by the government,[27] which we will discuss in more detail later on. Unless you are an elite athlete or in training for an event such as a marathon, eating additional protein after exercising is not something you need to do as long as you are eating some good-quality protein at each meal.

I'm told meat is a good source of protein, but isn't eating meat bad for me?

As we've established, few of us in the developed world are protein-deficient. The problem is that much of our protein intake comes with a large side order of saturated animal fat in the form of red meat. Apart from the ethical and sustainability issues surrounding meat consumption, a recent study found that eating meat at least three times a week was linked to a greater risk of nine different illnesses, including heart disease and diabetes.

Reducing our meat intake is a health no-brainer.[28] Indeed, current NHS guidelines advise cutting down to a mere 70g of meat per day, which is the equivalent of two rashers of bacon.[29] But how do we square this with getting enough protein, given that for most of us, meat is our main protein source?

Favouring leaner types of meat like chicken and turkey is a good idea, as well as sustainably caught or farmed fish and shellfish. Dairy products and eggs are also excellent sources of protein, and we should all be aiming to include more plant proteins in our diets, as these are cheaper and more sustainable than meat, and also provide additional gut-health benefits.

Are meat substitutes a healthy protein source?

Apart from natural plant proteins, there has been an explosion of plant-based meat alternatives on the market in the last few years. It's easy to assume that just because something is plant-based, it's automatically good for you. This is referred to as the 'health-halo' effect and has been ruthlessly exploited by food manufacturers. But it simply is not the case.

Fake meats market themselves on their health credentials, but these products are in fact classed as UPFs (ultra-processed foods) and can have high levels of saturated fat, sugar and salt. Indeed, here are the contents of a well-known brand of plant-based burger:

> Water, Pea Protein (16%), Rapeseed Oil, Coconut Oil, Rice Protein, Flavouring, Stabiliser (Methyl Cellulose), Potato Starch, Apple Extract, Colour (Beetroot Red), Maltodextrin, Pomegranate Extract, Salt, Potassium Chloride, Concentrated Lemon Juice, Maize Vinegar, Carrot Powder, Emulsifier (Sunflower Lecithin).

There's a lot going on there. Admittedly, they do provide considerable amounts of protein, but from a purely nutritional perspective, where we are aiming to minimise the amount of heavily processed foods in our diet, they aren't the best choice.

Why are plant proteins important?

Our diets tend to be skewed in favour of protein from animal sources, but researchers at Harvard University calculated that getting 3% more of their total calories in the form of plant protein (like beans, nuts and wholegrains) lowered people's risk for premature death by 5%.[30]

As we've discussed, most plant proteins are not 'complete' proteins, and so it's best to eat a range of different plant proteins to ensure adequate nutrition. There are some exceptions, however: soy, quinoa and chia seeds are complete proteins, so these are good ones to have in your kitchen cupboard.

What about protein powders?

Protein powders have taken off in the last few years as the trendy way to shoehorn extra protein into your diet, but it's important to note that although they do obviously contain protein, most don't have the additional vitamins and minerals that other protein-rich foods like nuts and pulses do.

However, a good-quality protein powder (without added sweeteners) can be a quick way to include protein in your meal, especially at breakfast time. Adding a couple of scoops to a morning smoothie will tick the protein box. This is useful for people on restrictive diets, for example vegans for whom animal proteins are off-limits, or those recovering from an injury or surgery who may need a temporary protein boost.

Is it possible to have too much protein?

Much of the discussion around protein focuses on 'getting enough'; indeed, the protein powders we've been discussing were created based on the notion that the more protein we can cram into our diets, the better. It's ironic given that protein deficiency is rare, and what is perhaps more surprising is that so little is said about the potential dangers of high-protein diets.

There isn't enough data for an upper 'safe' limit on protein consumption to have been set in the UK, but it's generally accepted that anything up to double the RNI – see below – is OK. It's simply worth being aware that if you are on a very high-protein diet, there are some risks, such as kidney damage from dehydration and calcium loss.

What are the best sources of protein, and how much should I eat?

According to the British Nutrition Foundation, the current RNI in the UK is 0.75g of protein per kilogram of bodyweight per day for adults, with additional requirements for growth and repair. For the 'average' woman, this means around 45g of protein a day; for men, it's around 55g. This can be hard to visualise on the plate, but as long as you are eating some protein at each meal, you are probably getting enough. The recipes later in the book state how many grams of each macronutrient they contain, which is useful when it comes to understanding portion size and how much protein to consume.

These are the best sources of protein, along with a guide to appropriate portion sizes:

Animal proteins

Fish – Sustainably caught or farmed fish and seafood provide plenty of protein and also those all-important omega-3 fatty acids. Aim to eat sustainable oily fish, like sardines, herring and mackerel, once a week; otherwise, choose white fish like pollock, coley or hake, farmed salmon and shrimp with the Aquaculture Stewardship Logo, and British crab and mussels.

Portion size – use the rule of palm. The piece of fish should be roughly the same size as the palm of your hand. Most types of fish and shellfish provide approximately 18–20g of protein per 100g.

Poultry – Free-range or organic (if you can afford it) chicken and turkey with the skin removed before eating offer a good way to get a protein hit with less saturated fat.

Portion size – use the rule of palm. The piece of chicken or turkey should be roughly the same size as the palm of your hand. Chicken or turkey provides approximately 30g of protein per 100g.

Lean cuts of red meat – Choose cuts of red meat with less than 10g total fat. This is usually specified on the packet. The leanest cuts are pork tenderloin, lean sirloin steak (or fillet steak, but this is pricey) and diced, lean lamb leg meat for use in curries and tagines.

Portion size – use the rule of palm. The piece of meat should be roughly the same size as the palm of your hand. Red meat provides approximately 25g of protein per 100g.

Eggs – Eggs are fabulous, protein-rich nutrition bombs. Food-wise, they are one of the best ways to start the day.

Portion size – 1 egg (6g protein).

Dairy – Dairy products like cheese and yogurt are protein-rich and convenient, the perfect choice for snacking. Cheese can be quite calorific, so if you are trying to lose weight, watch your portion size or stick to lower-calorie options, like cottage cheese, goat's cheese, feta and mozzarella. With yogurt, choose unsweetened live yogurt; you can always add fresh fruit and a drizzle of honey to sweeten.

Portion size – around 30g cheese (8g protein), 3 tablespoons cottage cheese (5g protein), 100g natural yogurt (5g protein).

Plant proteins

Soy foods – There has been some controversy around soy products, with the suggestion that they may be linked to a high risk of breast cancer and concerns around GMOs (commercially produced soy beans are often genetically modified). There is no strong scientific evidence to support these concerns, and soy remains one of the best complete plant proteins you can eat. Soy foods include miso, tofu, tempeh and edamame beans.

 Portion size – 75g edamame beans (13g protein), 100g tofu (17g protein).

Legumes – Legumes is the umbrella term for beans, peas, chickpeas, lentils, etc. You can buy them dried, tinned or in pre-cooked pouches for maximum convenience. They are one of the cheapest and most sustainable ways to eat protein. Combine them with other plant proteins to make sure you are getting the full range of amino acids.

 Portion size – 80g or 3 heaped tablespoons (6–8g protein) of cooked legumes.

Grains – Quinoa and buckwheat are your go-to here, as they are complete plant proteins, but all wholegrains are good protein sources, including oats and wholegrain rice. You can buy pouches of pre-cooked grain mixes. These are an excellent base for salads, or you can heat them up and add herbs and spices for a quick side dish.

 Portion size – 100g of cooked grains (4.5–5.5g protein).

Nuts and seeds – Nuts and seeds are extremely healthy sources of protein, and they can be added to all manner of dishes. Include them in porridge or overnight oats, sprinkle over eggs and on salads, add to bakes and cakes, or simply create your own healthy seed-and-nut snack mix. One good tip is to toast some chopped nuts and seeds in a pan so they are crunchy and keep in an airtight container to provide additional crunchy texture to meals. Don't forget chia and hemp seeds are also complete proteins.

 Portion size – 30g nuts (6g protein), 1 tablespoon seeds (2g protein).

Protein recap

- Protein is an important macronutrient for muscle growth and repair, hormone production and a robust immune system.
- Animal sources of protein contain all nine essential amino acids our bodies require, while most plant proteins (apart from a few, such as soy, quinoa and chia seeds) are incomplete and should be eaten in combination.
- It's a good idea to limit protein intake from red meat, which can be high in saturated fat, and try to get more from leaner animal and plant sources Don't be tempted to replace with fake meats, which are highly processed foods.
- Protein powders can be useful for those on restricted diets or for those needing an additional protein boost.
- The average person needs around 45–55g of protein a day. While there is no agreed safe upper limit for protein intake, it's worth noting that there are some risks associated with very high-protein diets.
- The best sources of protein are sustainable seafood, lean meat, eggs, dairy, soy, legumes, grains, nuts and seeds.

Ten easy ways to focus on lean and plant proteins

1. **Have some protein at every meal.** For example, eggs, oats or yogurt at breakfast time, some beans or fish for lunch, such as a tuna and bean salad, and some grilled fish or lean meat with wholegrains for dinner.

2. **Add a protein powder to your smoothie.** If you are lactose intolerant or vegan, then getting protein into a smoothie can be tricky. A scoop or two of protein powder can help, but do check the ingredients and make sure there is no added sugar. If you eat dairy, then try adding cottage cheese instead – see the Protein Power Smoothie on page 136.

3. **Combine your plant proteins.** Eat different plant proteins in combination to make sure you are getting all the different amino acids: for example, try overnight oats with a mixture of grains, nuts and seeds, like the Ten-plant-foods Overnight Oats on page 179.

4. **Eat more 'everyday' legumes.** Did you know that garden peas, green beans, sugar snap peas and mangetout are all protein-rich legumes? Another legume you probably also already eat regularly is the humble baked bean, as are peanuts, which make an excellent snack.

5. **Have tins of beans, chickpeas and lentils handy.** Use in salads, add to family favourites like Bolognese sauce, cottage pie, curries and stews, or try something new, like the Mushroom and Lentil Masala recipe on page 140.

6. **Have some hummus.** Most of us have a pot of hummus in the fridge, and it's an excellent protein-rich snack. Enjoy on some wholegrain crackers or cut up some veggie sticks for dipping.

7. **Stock up the freezer with peas, broad beans and edamame beans.** Frozen peas and beans are not just convenient, they are surprisingly high in protein, and because they are picked and frozen straight away, they often retain more of their vitamin and mineral content than fresh ones, which have had a long journey to the supermarket.

8. **Experiment with seafood.** Seafood is a great source of protein, but this doesn't just mean fish. Try and broaden your

horizons to include more shellfish, like sustainable British crab. Try the Crab Guacamole Toast-topper on page 205.

9. **Eat some lean meat each week.** This is advisable, not just for the protein it contains, but also for iron, vitamin B12 and zinc. Choose leaner cuts like pork tenderloin – try the Sweet and Sour Pork Tenderloin with Braised Cabbage on page 146.

10. **Try different types of soy.** Miso, tofu and edamame beans are quite commonplace these days, but another soy ingredient you may be less familiar with is tempeh. This is fermented soy beans that come in a firm block, which you can then slice and use in place of meat in curries and stews. To get started, try the Indonesian Vegetables and Tempeh in a Coconut Milk Broth on page 188.

THREE

Include Healthy Fats

What is fat, and why do I need it?

If you are over 40, you belong to the low-fat generation, hard-wired to reach for the skimmed milk, low-fat spread or fat-free yogurt. For decades, the advice was to reduce fat, especially saturated animal fat, in our diets, and so we came to fear it, imagining our arteries clogging up as we tucked into a juicy steak. But dietary fat is a key macronutrient essential to good health.

The main role of fat in the body is to provide energy and support cell function. Fat also helps your body absorb some nutrients, in particular the fat-soluble vitamins A, D, E and K. It is also important in hormone production.

There are four types of dietary fat, each with different chemical structures and physical properties:

Monounsaturated fats – These are considered the healthiest fats, because they help reduce blood cholesterol, blood pressure and other heart-disease risk factors. Sources include olive oil, rapeseed oil, avocados and some nuts and seeds.

Polyunsaturated fats – These are a type of healthy fat that includes omega-3 and omega-6 fatty acids, which are essential for brain function. They are present in oily fish, vegetable oils, nuts and seeds.

Saturated fats – Saturated fats are usually solid at room temperature and common in animal products like meat and dairy, and tropical oils like coconut oil and palm oil.

Trans fats – Trans fats are vegetable oils that have been industrially manipulated to make them more saturated and semi-solid at room temperature. They are inexpensive and widely used in the production of processed foods.

But isn't eating fat bad for the heart?

Well, yes and no. The real baddies here are the trans fats, which go by lots of different names, such as 'partially hydrogenated oil' or 'mono and diglycerides of fatty acids', so it's really important to check the ingredients labels of the products you buy regularly. Many studies have linked trans fats to an increased risk of heart disease, and they should be avoided if at all possible.[31]

While the UK government has encouraged food manufacturers to reduce the levels of trans fats in products, an outright ban has yet to be brought in. Moreover, there is no legal requirement in the UK for companies to place warning labels on foods that contain trans fats. Currently, the best way to avoid trans fats is to avoid processed foods.

There has also been much debate around the role saturated animal fat plays in increasing the risk of cardiovascular disease, and it is often lumped in as a 'bad' fat along with trans fats. The evidence is far from conclusive. A 2020 review of various studies found that the association between the two appears to be very weak.[32] Notwithstanding this, saturated animal fat doesn't provide many nutritional benefits, other than energy, which is best gained from other healthier sources.

Conversely, monounsaturated fat can be very heart-healthy, in particular the nutritional all-star, olive oil. A recent study found that overweight and obese people who followed a diet lower in carbohydrates and higher in healthy fats saw improvements in their risk factors for cardiovascular disease not related to weight loss.[33]

This pushes back against the previous low-fat doctrine and supports the idea that a diet containing good fats is indeed heart-healthy, but it must be emphasised that the overall quality of the diet is key.

Munching through cheese-laden takeaway pizza is not going to do your heart any favours, but making olive oil your choice of fat in the kitchen will.

What's the deal with cholesterol?

Cholesterol is one of the most misunderstood areas of nutrition. There are actually two types of blood cholesterol: HDL, which is often called the 'good' cholesterol, and LDL, the 'bad' one. Both are kinds of fatty acid that circulate in the blood and are non-essential, meaning our bodies can make what we need, although we do also consume cholesterol via animal products such as meat and eggs.

Cholesterol is used to build our cell walls, to make bile acids to digest fat in the intestine and in the production of vitamin D and hormones. The problem comes when there's too much LDL cholesterol in the blood, as it can be deposited in the arteries, increasing the risk of heart problems. HDL, on the other hand, gathers up excess cholesterol and deposits it in the liver to be turned into bile, so a healthy diet aims to increase HDL and reduce LDL.

To be clear, diet is only one factor here; there are other lifestyle risk factors that can affect this balance, including smoking, exercise, body weight, alcohol and salt intake.

If I eat fat won't I put on weight?

A famous actress once said, 'If you don't eat fat, you won't get fat,' which is proof enough that we shouldn't take nutritional advice from celebrities! It seems logical on the face of it, but fat is just one of the three macronutrients that provide energy, and it's your overall energy balance that determines if you put on weight or not (in the absence of other medical factors, of course).

So, the simple answer to this question is no, but there's a little more to it than that: 1g of fat delivers nine calories, whereas

1g of protein or carbohydrates has just four calories. Added to this, of the three macronutrients, fat has the lowest thermic effect, which means it takes the least amount of energy to digest. To put it another way, you burn fewer calories digesting fat than you do carbohydrates and protein. What this means in practice is that the relative portion size of higher-fat foods should be smaller than the other two macronutrients.

What is omega-3 and why do I need it?

Omega-3s are a family of essential fatty acids that play important roles in the body and may provide a number of health benefits, in particular reducing the risk of cardiovascular disease.

The three most important types are ALA (alpha-linolenic acid), DHA (docosahexaenoic acid), and EPA (eicosapentaenoic acid). ALA is mainly found in plants, while DHA and EPA occur mostly in animal foods, in particular oily fish and algae.

It's important to note that ALA needs to be converted into DHA and EPA in order to be useful to the body, but our systems are pretty inefficient at making this conversion. Any ALA that is not converted is simply used as energy, like other fats. Plant-based forms of omega-3 do have a role to play, but for maximum benefit, we need to include foods containing DHA and EPA in our diets.

Should I take an omega-3 supplement?

Fish oil supplements are nothing new. Indeed, bottles of cod liver oil were given out by the Ministry of Food during and after the Second World War when rationing was in place, as a way to support the nation's nutrition. Today, omega-3 supplements are big business, with the global market expected to reach $4.86 billion USD by 2028.

The craze for omega-3 began in the 1980s, when a spate of studies were published linking omega-3 intake with better long-term health outcomes across a range of conditions. Over the past ten years, more than 12,500 scientific studies on the benefits of omega-3 have been published, so it's easy to see why consumers feel it's better to be safe than sorry and pop another tub of capsules in the shopping trolley.

However, the British Dietetic Association (BDA) doesn't recommend omega-3 supplements for the general population, because the evidence of their benefits is inconclusive.[34] Instead, they advise us to focus on getting the omega-3 we need from our food. That's not to say supplements don't deliver any benefits, and there may be scenarios when supplements are advisable, for example if you have children who are picky eaters and don't like fish, or if you are following a restricted diet for ethical or medical reasons.

If you choose to take an omega-3 supplement, the advice from the BDA is as follows:

- Check the vitamin A content of the supplement. You should not have more than a total of 1.5mg vitamin A (1500ug) a day from food and supplements combined.

- Choose omega-3 rather than fish liver oil, as the latter can contain very high levels of vitamin A.

- Do not take supplements containing vitamin A if you are pregnant or planning to become pregnant.

- Check the label for DHA and EPA content, and choose a supplement that provides you with the same daily amount you would get from eating one to two portions of fish per week (about 450mg EPA and DHA per daily adult dose).

- Choose an age-appropriate supplement – children will need less than adults.

- Vegans and vegetarians can take an EPA and DHA supplement derived from marine algae.

What about omega-6?

You may have heard of omega-6, another essential dietary fat that is found mainly in refined cooking oils, especially soy bean, sunflower and corn oils. Having too much omega-6 in the diet can increase the risk of inflammation and inflammatory conditions. The key thing to note here is that it's the ratio between the amounts of omega-3 and omega-6 you are eating that has health implications.

Scientists have suggested that a diet high in omega-6s but low in omega-3s increases inflammation, while a diet that includes balanced amounts of each reduces inflammation.[35] The way to decrease your omega-6 intake is to switch to oils that contain less of it, like rapeseed and olive oil, and to avoid processed foods, where oils high in omega-6 are commonly used.

What are the best sources of healthy fat and how much should I eat?

The government recommends that total fat intake should not exceed 35% of our daily calorie intake, and saturated fat intake should not exceed 11%, which is roughly 30g per day for men and 20g per day for women.[36] This is tricky to understand in the context of the food on our plates, as we can't easily visualise it.

The best approach is to focus on eating healthy fats and minimising the unhealthy fats rather than obsessing over the exact quantity. You'll find that if you are consuming a decent amount of healthy fat, it goes a long way towards regulating appetite and you will be less likely to overeat. As discussed previously, however, fat is the most calorific of the three macronutrients, so for very high-fat foods, it is worth having an understanding of appropriate portion sizes (see below).

As far as omega-3 intake goes, there is no official RNI in the UK, and little general consensus on the optimal amount to include in our diets. In the USA, they suggest 1.6g per day for an adult, but here in the UK the advice is more general and amounts to eating one 140g portion of oily fish weekly and including plenty of healthy plant sources of omega-3, such as walnuts, chia seeds and flaxseeds.

Animal sources

Oily fish – Oily fish is the best food source of omega-3, and it is currently recommended that you eat some once a week. Choose sustainable species that are further down the food chain, such as sardines, herring and anchovies. Other good options are line-caught mackerel and rainbow trout. Salmon is the most popular oily fish in the UK, but be sure to look for sustainably caught/farmed versions.
Portion size – 140g (18g fat, 291 calories).

Eggs – For a long time, it was thought that because egg yolks contain a fair amount of cholesterol, they increased blood cholesterol levels, and that our consumption should be limited to one or two eggs a week. Current thinking is that the impact on blood cholesterol has been over-egged – no pun intended – and that for most people, eating one to two a day is fine because of the other health benefits they confer.[37]
Portion size – 1 egg (5g fat, 75 calories).

Dairy – The latest advice coming through supports choosing full-fat versions of dairy products rather than low-fat, as full-fat versions don't seem to increase the risk of heart disease as previously thought.[38] Also, full-fat versions are usually less processed and less likely to contain unwanted ingredients that have been added to replace the fat. Sticking to sensible portion sizes means that you won't be consuming too many calories.
Portion size – 30g cheese (10g fat, 121 calories); 100g full-fat unsweetened Greek yogurt (9g fat, 117 calories); 1 teaspoon butter (4g fat, 34 calories).

Plant sources

Avocados – While there are some ethical issues around global avocado production, they are one of the healthiest plant-based sources of fat. They are also rich in antioxidants, potassium and fibre, and studies have shown they can have favourable effects on blood cholesterol levels.[39]

Portion size – ¼ avocado (8g fat, 80 calories).

Nuts – Not only are nuts bursting with healthy fats, but studies have shown that people who eat nuts regularly tend to be healthier overall and have a lower risk of various diseases, including heart disease and type 2 diabetes.[40] Just a word of caution, though: they are pretty heavy on the calories, so be sure to eat no more than the recommended portion size of a small handful or 30g per day.

Portion size – 30g almonds (15g fat, 173 calories); 30g cashews (13g fat, 166 calories); 30g walnuts (19g fat, 196 calories).

Seeds – Seeds are an excellent source of monounsaturated and polyunsaturated fats in the diet, particularly the plant-based form of omega-3 fatty acid ALA. Try and include some in your diet every day.

Portion size – 1 tablespoon sunflower seeds (4.5g fat, 51 calories); 1 tablespoon pumpkin seeds (4g fat, 45 calories); 1 tablespoon flaxseeds (4.5g fat, 55 calories); 1 tablespoon chia seeds (4g fat, 58 calories).

Oils – When it comes to oils, the rule of thumb is to choose a high-smoke point oil for cooking and use unrefined/cold-pressed oils for flavouring. Olive oil is the healthiest choice; for cooking, use the light-coloured version, and for drizzling and dressings, use good-quality extra virgin. When you need a neutral oil for high-temperature cooking like frying, a good choice is rapeseed oil, preferably organic.

Portion size – 1 tablespoon (14g fat, 120 calories).

Healthy fats recap

- Fat is an important macronutrient used in many of the body's processes, as well as for providing energy and enabling the absorption of the fat-soluble vitamins A, D, E and K.
- The healthiest fats are the monounsaturated ones found in olive oil, avocados, and some nuts and seeds, and the omega-3 fatty acids found in oily fish, chia seeds, flaxseeds and walnuts.
- For heart health, avoid trans fats, often found in processed foods, and eat saturated fats in moderation.
- Cholesterol is a kind of fat found in animal products that has been linked to heart disease. For this reason, those at risk should limit saturated animal fat in their diets, but other lifestyle factors are equally important in keeping cholesterol levels under control.
- Omega-6 is a kind of fat that should be reduced in favour of omega-3. It is especially high in soy bean, corn and sunflower oils.
- Fat is the most calorific of the three macronutrients, so if you are trying to lose weight, it's important to keep an eye on portion size.

Ten easy ways to incorporate healthy fats

1. **Switch to full-fat dairy products.** The myth that full-fat dairy products are bad for the heart has been debunked, and less-processed, full-fat dairy products not only taste better, but they are also more satiating and so help with appetite control. Ditch flavoured yogurts and buy full-fat Greek yogurt instead. Full-fat

cheese is fine in moderation, and butter is better than low-fat spreads, but use sparingly as it is calorific.

2. **Don't be afraid of eggs.** Despite past bad press, eating one to two a day delivers not only healthy fats but a whole range of nutrients and protein. Omelettes are back on! Try the Prawn and Pak Choy Omelette on page 137.

3. **Be selective with meat.** When it comes to meat, it still makes sense to choose lean cuts and remove any visible fat. Buy minced meat with 5% fat and trim any excess fat off bacon and steaks. Pork tenderloin and skinless chicken and turkey are good choices.

4. **Eat mainly plant fats.** Plant fats are among the healthiest you can eat, especially those intrinsic to whole foods like avocados, nuts and seeds. But be calorie-aware: a portion size for avocado is just a quarter of a fruit, while 14 almonds are 100 calories, as is 1 tablespoon of peanut butter.

5. **Sort out your oils.** Use organic rapeseed oil or light olive oil for cooking and extra virgin olive oil for drizzling and dressings as your kitchen standards.

6. **Make your own salad dressings.** Commercial salad dressings are often high in unhealthy fat or added sugars. Create your own dressings with olive, flaxseed or sesame oils.

7. **Eat oily fish once a week for omega-3.** Declining fish stocks are a global issue, so it's best to choose sustainable varieties such as rainbow trout, herring and mackerel. Tinned oily fish like sardines and anchovies, where you eat the bones, are particularly good, because you also get a big hit of calcium. A great recipe to get a sustainable omega-3 fix is the Pan-fried Rainbow Trout with Mushrooms and Chard on page 212.

8. **Eat more plant-based sources of omega-3.** Although not as bioavailable as the omega-3 found in oily fish, plant sources

of omega-3, such as chia seeds, flaxseeds and walnuts, are still a useful addition to the diet. Make some of the Omega-3 Nut Butter on page 151 and have a little every day, either spread on apple slices or stuffed into a pitted date for a healthy snack.

9. **Balance your omega-3 and omega-6.** Fresh soy products like edamame and tofu, while they do contain some omega-6, are considered very healthy because of all the other benefits they provide. Edamame and oily fish go extremely well together, and this is a good example of balancing omega-3 and omega-6 in the diet. Try the Wild Salmon Poke Bowl (page 142), which contains both.

10. **Switch to high-cocoa-solids chocolate.** Dark chocolate (over 85%) contains over 65% fat, which is mostly oleic acid (a heart-healthy fat also found in olive oil), as well as a range of nutrients and antioxidants. The portion size is just one to two squares, though, as the calorie load is quite high.

FOUR

Have 30g of Fibre a Day

What is fibre, and why does my body need it?

It keeps you regular! That's the one thing I knew about fibre even before I became interested in health, possibly something to do with those old All-Bran adverts. And, indeed, it does, but as well as keeping our bowels moving and our gut bacteria fed, fibre also plays an important role in weight management by regulating our appetites and slowing down digestion so that blood sugar levels are more consistent.

Fibre is, in simple terms, a type of carbohydrate that the body cannot digest, and it comes in two forms, soluble and insoluble:

Soluble fibre – As the name suggests, soluble fibre can absorb water and in doing so, it forms a gel in our stomachs. With a belly full of jelly we feel fuller (the appetite regulation mentioned above). It can also bind to cholesterol in the gut, preventing it from being absorbed into the blood stream, good for those looking to reduce their cholesterol markers. Legumes, wholegrains, cruciferous vegetables like broccoli and sprouts and citrus fruit are high in soluble fibre.

Insoluble fibre – Yep, you've guessed it: this type of fibre doesn't absorb water, and it effectively works like a big brush, moving through the gut and removing old cells and debris. An intestinal chimney sweep, if you like. This type of fibre is also sometimes called roughage, and it not only makes us feel fuller, it also prevents constipation. It is found in wholegrains and fruits and vegetables, particularly in the skins.

There is a third type of fibre, which, confusingly, isn't called fibre at all. Resistant starch has characteristics of both insoluble and soluble fibre, in that it 'resists' digestion, but once in the large intestine it ferments and feeds the good bacteria. Gut-friendly foods containing resistant starch are also referred to as prebiotics and include underripe bananas, garlic, onions, asparagus and cooked and cooled rice.

If fibre is a carbohydrate, why is it recommended to help prevent diabetes?

It's true, we usually associate type 2 diabetes with an over-consumption of carbs, or more specifically simple carbohydrates (remember those free sugars?). So how can eating fibre, also a carbohydrate, help reduce that risk?

The important thing to remember is that fibre is a type of carbohydrate *that the body can't digest*, and so it doesn't impact directly on blood sugar levels in the way that simple carbohydrates do. We also saw that fibre plays an import role in slowing down digestion, which in turn slows the release of glucose into the blood, and it's those blood sugar spikes that eventually lead to insulin resistance.

A recent study review looking at the role higher-fibre diets play in diabetes control concluded that 'higher-fibre diets are an important component of diabetes management, resulting in improvements in measures of glycaemic control, blood lipids, body weight, and inflammation, as well as a reduction in premature mortality'.[41]

These impacts of fibre in the diet are something we can all benefit from, not just those at risk of diabetes.

Won't eating too much fibre make me bloated and gassy?

Not to put too fine a point on it, but fibre makes you fart. As we've seen, part of the role of fibre is to ferment and feed the good bacteria in our guts. A by-product of this process is gas, namely hydrogen, methane and carbon dioxide.

Bloating and excess gas are usually caused by consuming too much fibre in one sitting, or, if you are trying to increase the fibre in your diet, by doing it too quickly. If you do experience any of these unwanted side-effects, try increasing your water intake and see if that helps (see below for some hydration tips). If not, then it might be time to dial down the fibre-rich foods. This can be a problem, particularly for vegans and vegetarians, whose diets may contain lots of legumes, fruit and vegetables.

It's also worth noting that having too much fibre can cause nutrient deficiencies, as it can interfere with the body's ability to absorb essential nutrients, such as calcium, magnesium, zinc and iron. As with most things when it comes to nutrition, balance is key.

Stay hydrated

In order for fibre to do its work, it draws water into the bowel, so you may become dehydrated if you do not drink enough. If you struggle to remember to drink water, here are some helpful hydration tips:

- Link having a glass of water to certain activities – have one with your morning tea or coffee, one before each meal, and one after exercising, for example.
- Set alerts on your phone or download one of the many apps that will notify you when it's time to have a drink.
- Eat hydrating foods, such as watermelon, berries, peaches, cucumber, lettuce, courgettes, celery, tomatoes and red peppers. Dairy products, including milk, yogurt and cottage cheese, are also good sources of water.

Can eating a fibre-rich diet help with weight loss?

Simply eating more fibre with no other interventions won't necessarily lead to weight loss. To lose weight, your system has to be in an energy deficit; in other words, it needs to be using more energy than it is taking in, and that is down to how much you are eating overall, as well as your exercise levels and other biological factors like your basal metabolic rate.

Let's not forget, however, that fibre plays an important role in appetite control, so eating more fibre may help you to feel less hungry, which will in turn lead to you consuming fewer calories. Fibre is also good for the gut, and if your microbiome is firing on all cylinders, it will help you process your food efficiently. This all feeds into that all-important energy-balance equation.

So, while eating fibre doesn't directly make you lose weight, it does help create the conditions where weight loss is more achievable.

What about 'added fibre' in foods – is this beneficial in the same way?

You may have noticed products on the supermarket shelves claiming to contain 'added fibre', and it's these kind of marketing triggers that play on our diet insecurities and have us filling our trolley with highly processed foods.

So what *is* added fibre, and can it help us increase our fibre intake? Added fibre can be synthetic or derived from natural sources – things like polydextrose, pectin, guar gum and cellulose are commonly found in products in the UK. While these things are considered safe to eat, the benefits of added fibre as compared to the fibre found in whole foods is unclear.

What we do know is that the unhealthy nature of most processed foods (in the case of fibre, these are often in the form of high-sugar cereal bars or breakfast cereals) probably negates the benefits of any additional fibre you may be getting. Synthetic fibre in particular does not offer the vitamins and minerals found in foods naturally high in fibre.

Rather than purchasing processed foods with added fibre, it's easy to add extra fibre to your meals at home. See 'Ten easy ways to eat 30g fibre a day' on page 61 for some ideas on how to do this.

What are the best sources of fibre, and how much should I eat?

The recommended daily intake of fibre for an adult is 30g, but according to the Food and Drink Federation, only a paltry 9% of adults in the UK are getting enough.[42] They also make the important point that government policy focuses very much on reducing the amount of calories, salt and sugar we consume, but there has been little focus on increasing the foods and nutrients we need more of, like fibre.

Admittedly, it can be difficult to visualise what 30g of fibre looks like when it comes to the food on our plate, so here are a few easy ways to fill up on fibre:

Wholegrains – Grains have three parts: the bran, the germ and the endosperm. Wholegrains are simply grains that have all three parts intact, unlike refined grains, which are stripped of valuable nutrients during the refining process. Wholegrains have lots of insoluble fibre, as well as iron, magnesium, manganese, phosphorus, selenium and B vitamins. The best sources are wholegrain bread, wholegrain cereal, wholemeal pasta, oats and brown rice.

Portion size – 1 large slice (40g) of wholegrain bread (3g fibre); 55g of fibre-rich muesli – see page 163 (12g fibre); 75g (uncooked weight) wholemeal pasta (7.5g fibre); 40g oats (8.5g fibre); 75g (uncooked weight) brown rice (3g fibre).

Fruit – There are many fibre-rich fruits, and packaged up with the fibre are lots of micronutrients, too, so snacking on fruit ticks a lot of nutritional boxes. Berries are particularly good because they also contain antioxidant polyphenols and are naturally low in calories.

Portion size – 50g raspberries (4g fibre); 1 pear (6g fibre); 1 medium-sized banana (3g fibre); 1 apple (4.5g fibre).

Nuts – As well as being packed with nutrients and healthy fats, nuts are full of fibre too. Almonds, pistachios and hazelnuts are particularly fibre-rich.

Portion size – 30g almonds (3.5g fibre); 30g pistachios (3g fibre); 30g hazelnuts (3g fibre).

Fibre recap

- Fibre is a type of carbohydrate the body can't digest. It helps keep the gut and bowels healthy, and helps regulate appetite and blood sugar levels.
- Fibre lowers the risk of developing type 2 diabetes by slowing digestion. This prevents blood sugar spikes, which can lead to insulin resistance over time.
- Most of us don't eat enough fibre, but having too much can cause gas and bloating. If you experience this, reduce your fibre intake and keep hydrated.
- Fibre creates favourable conditions for weight loss by increasing satiety (the sense of feeling full after eating), which reduces appetite and subsequent calorie intake.
- Avoid processed products with added fibre. Instead, increase the amount of fibre in your meals and snacks.
- The recommended intake for an adult is 30g of fibre per day. The best sources are wholegrains, fruit, nuts, legumes and potatoes in their skins.

Legumes – Beans, peas and lentils are all excellent sources of fibre, and in particular the fermentable fibre that our gut bacteria love to feast on.

Portion size – ½ can of mixed beans (8.5g fibre); 80g frozen peas (5g fibre); 100g cooked lentils (8g fibre).

Potatoes – You don't need to go too off-piste in order to increase the fibre in your diet. Potatoes with their skins on are full of fibre, and they also contain a helpful hit of vitamin C.

Portion size – 1 medium potato with the skin on (5g fibre).

Ten easy ways to eat 30g fibre a day

1. **Switch to wholegrains.** Change to buying exclusively wholegrain bread, brown rice and wholemeal pasta.

2. **Use cooked and cooled rice pouches for resistant starch.** You can add these to soups (see Kedgeree Soup on page 153) and salads, or mix with fresh herbs and spices for an instant side dish.

3. **Seek out psyllium husk.** This is a brilliant way to add fibre to smoothies, porridge, pancakes and bakes. If you can't find it in your supermarket, you can buy it online.

4. **Buy or make some nut butter.** Nut butters are a great source of fibre, particularly when paired with wholegrain bread. Try the Omega-3 Nut Butter on page 151.

5. **Make your own cereals for breakfast.** Don't buy shop-bought cereals, which are high in sugar. Instead, make your own Fibre-rich Muesli (see page 163) or Wholegrain Granola (see page 122). Top with fresh berries for extra fibre.

6. **Stock up on cans of beans.** Beans are your fibre friend, especially black beans, which also contain loads of antioxidants. They can be added to soups, curries and stews – or try making the Smoky Black Bean, Aubergine and Red Pepper Tortillas on page 174.

7. **Don't forget good old baked beans.** Pile half a tin on to a thick slice of wholegrain toast, and you will get a whopping 11g fibre.

8. **Learn to love lentils.** Lentils are a brilliant plant-based source of protein and fibre, and are extremely versatile. There are two fabulous lentil recipes in the fibre section later in the book, Lentil Shakshouka on page 164 and Everyday Dal on page 170.

9. **Have a cracker snack.** Hummus on wholegrain crackers is a filling and fibre-rich snack you can eat at any time of the day.

10. **Eat the skins.** Leave the skins on potatoes when you bake, roast or boil them. For mash, boil with the skins on and lightly crush; you can add a little Greek yogurt and chopped spring onion for flavour instead of butter.

FIVE

Support Your Gut Health

What is a healthy gut?

The human body is host to a vast number of microbes, which together constitute what is known as our microbiota. Most of these reside in the small intestine and colon – the microbiome – and are essential to many aspects of our health and well-being. Gut microbes perform a number of functions; as well as absorbing energy and nutrients from our food, they can also influence our food cravings and have a role in signalling when we are full.

While there is no official definition of what constitutes a 'healthy gut', there are certain attributes of the microbiome that are associated with good gut health:

Richness/diversity – Richness refers to the total number of bacterial species present in the gut microbiome, and diversity is the number of individual bacteria from each of the bacterial species.

Stability – A stable microbiome is one that is resistant to factors that can potentially disrupt the microbiota, including genetic factors, dietary modifications, age and various medications.

Resilience – A resilient microbiome quickly returns to a healthy state after a disturbance, for example after antibiotic treatment.

Why is a healthy gut so important?

Not a week goes by without a new study confirming the critical role our gut bacteria play in our overall health. Many lifestyle and environmental factors contribute to our gut health. Diet is obviously key, but whether we smoke, how much we exercise, our quality of sleep and our stress levels can all have an impact.

There are three main ways that our microbiomes keep our minds and bodies healthy:

Weight management – The make-up of your gut bacteria affects how your food is digested, how fat is stored and whether you feel hungry or full. A healthy gut, therefore, creates better conditions for maintaining a healthy weight, which in turn lowers the risk of chronic diseases such as cancer and heart disease.

Mind and mood – The vagus nerve connects the brain and the gut, creating a biological pathway known as the gut–brain axis. Evidence is mounting that this relationship has a significant impact on our mental well-being. A 2017 study in Australia called the SMILES Trial set out to study the impact of dietary improvement for people suffering with moderate to severe depression. Participants were either placed on a supervised Mediterranean-style diet or received counselling with no dietary intervention. At the end of the trial, 30% of those in the dietary intervention group met the criteria for remission of major depression, compared to just 8% of those who had received counselling only.[43] Although the study didn't look specifically at the microbiome composition, it's well known that this way of eating (wholegrains, fruit and veg, legumes, good-quality dairy, raw and unsalted nuts, fish, lean red meat, chicken, eggs and olive oil) has a positive impact on gut bacteria.

Immunity – Research is increasingly revealing a positive correlation between a diverse gut microbiome and a healthy immune system. In fact, it is estimated that around 70–80% of our immune cells are housed in the gut.[44] An immune system that is firing on all cylinders will not only be better able to fight off bugs and infection, it also reduces chronic inflammation, which can lead to diseases such as cancer and autoimmune conditions.

What are the best ways to support gut health?

Given the crucial role the microbiome plays in our overall health, what we eat needs to support good gut health. Thankfully, it's quite straightforward. It's important to eat more fibre and omega-3, as we've already covered, but the single best thing you can do for your gut health is to eat 30 different plant foods a week. Indeed, research from the American Gut Project backs this up,[45] and leading UK gut experts such as Professor Tim Spector and Dr Megan Rossi also support this advice.

It might seem a tall order, but it's important to remember that the term 'plant foods' includes not just fruit and vegetables, but grains and legumes, nuts and seeds, and herbs and spices. Other than getting your 30-a-week, here are a few other tips for a happy gut:

- Chew your food. Chewing is the first stage of digestion. When you thoroughly chew your food, the digestive enzymes can do their work more efficiently, which improves digestion and nutrient absorption.

- Eat foods rich in polyphenols. These are plant chemicals found in colourful fruit and vegetables, coffee, red wine, olive oil, and herbs and spices. They increase gut microbe diversity.

- Eat fermented foods like kimchi, kombucha, kefir and live yogurt, which are rich in gut-friendly probiotic bacteria.

- Avoid processed foods, which tend to contain trans fats and high levels of salt and free sugars, all of which negatively affect your gut bacteria.

Are there certain things I should cut out of my diet to help my gut health?

When people experience adverse gut symptoms, like bloating, their first instinct is to start cutting things out of their diet. Why? Because restrictive diets are big business, and billions of pounds have been pumped into marketing 'free-from' products that encourage eliminating certain foods – and, indeed, whole food groups – as the way to health nirvana.

The irony here, of course, is that for optimal gut health, the exact opposite is true. In the absence of any medical condition, intolerance or allergy, the absolute best advice is to have as inclusive a diet as possible. This doesn't extend, for obvious reasons, to include ultra-processed foods, which should be minimised; what we are talking about here is a varied, balanced, whole-food diet.

If you do experience bloating, stomach-cramping episodes, constipation or diarrhoea, the first line of defence is to support your gut health by following the tips given in this chapter and including plenty of gut-friendly foods. If you still have discomfort, then it's time to consult your GP. Gut-health issues are usually complex, so randomly cutting out foods or popping supplements to try and get to the bottom of the problem – no pun intended – is generally not the best approach.

But isn't gluten bad for the gut?

Gluten has had a bad rap over the last decade as the gluten-free movement has gained traction. But simply speaking, gluten is just a protein found in wheat, barley and rye, and for the vast majority of us, it can be eaten with no adverse effects. Indeed, wholegrain products are advised as part of a healthy, balanced diet, and are an important source of fibre.

A growing number of people are cutting gluten out of their diets for perceived health or weight-loss benefits, but unless you have one of the following conditions, there is absolutely no reason to cut out gluten:

Coeliac disease – This is an autoimmune disease caused by your body mistaking gluten for an alien invasion, much as if you had a virus, and producing antibodies to fight it. This causes damage to the gut lining, which leads to digestive problems, weight loss and fatigue, but can also lead to longer-term conditions, such as coronary artery disease and small bowel cancer. There is no cure for coeliac disease, and the only way to manage it is by following a completely gluten-free diet.

Gluten intolerance/sensitivity – Some people experience symptoms similar to coeliac disease after eating gluten but do not have the disease. There is no way to definitively diagnose an intolerance; it usually involves following an elimination diet under the supervision of a qualified dietitian. You cannot diagnose a gluten intolerance with a home-testing kit! Gluten intolerance is not thought to impact health in the longer term, unlike coeliac disease.

Wheat allergy – Here, it is wheat rather than specifically gluten that causes an allergic reaction when ingested. It can be life-threatening in severe cases, but more common symptoms include breathing difficulties, skin rashes, gut discomfort, a runny nose, sneezing and headaches. Wheat has to be completely eliminated from the diet. Rye and barley as well as other grains can usually still be eaten.

What is the FODMAP diet? I've heard it's good for people with gut problems.

The FODMAP diet was designed by researchers at Monash University in Australia as a temporary intervention diet to help people suffering with digestive disorders such as irritable bowel syndrome (IBS), a common condition that affects the digestive system causing stomach cramps, bloating, diarrhoea and constipation.

The diet works by eliminating foods containing FODMAPs, a collection of short-chain carbohydrates that can trigger IBS symptoms. FODMAPs are found naturally in many foods, such as wheat, garlic and onions, and in certain food additives.

The diet begins with a period of high restriction and then transitions to a more relaxed diet where foods are gradually reintroduced to identify which ones are troublesome. Despite including the word 'diet', a low-FODMAP approach to eating is not intended as a weight-loss plan. It's a very restrictive diet, and in order to be effective, it must be followed rigidly and under strict supervision.

Are regular cleanses and detoxes good for the gut?

In a word, no. As we've discussed, the gut likes variety, and cleanses and detoxes are, by their nature, restrictive. The body is perfectly capable of detoxing itself; that is, after all, what our liver, kidneys, lungs and skin are doing day in, day out. Far better to concentrate on eating a healthy, balanced diet including a wide variety of plant foods. This will do far more for your gut than you drinking juices for days on end.

Should I take a probiotic supplement?

We all know we need to pay more attention to our gut health, but the problem comes when busy lifestyles lead to poor food choices – grabbing food on the hoof is not the best way to nurture our good bacteria. We might, then, be tempted to resort to expensive supplements. Indeed, the market for probiotic products is worth around £750 million in the UK alone. But the efficacy of these products remains largely unproven.

What further complicates matters is that there are lots of different types of probiotics that all do different things in our bodies. Most people have no idea which of these they are deficient in, if at all. Taking a random probiotic is a bit like taking any other random supplement – it's a scattergun approach that is unlikely to hit the mark. By far the best way to improve gut health is via what we eat.

What is 'leaky gut syndrome', and do I need to worry about it?

The leakiness, or otherwise, of the gut refers to its permeability: in other words, how easy it is for material to pass from the gut into the blood stream. The implication here being that a leakier gut will let larger, potentially toxic molecules through.

Leaky gut is not, in itself, a condition, but the symptom of other factors. For example, coeliacs experience increased leakiness if they do not completely eliminate gluten, while drinking alcohol can temporarily increase the gut's permeability, as can stress. Once the underlying cause has been resolved, the gut should recover.

What are the best foods for gut health, and how much should I eat?

As we've already seen, eating a wide variety of plant foods is the key to a happy microbiome. There are also some other specific groups of foods that have been proven to support gut health. There's no recommended portion size as such for these foods in terms of RNI; the aim is merely to include some of these foods in your diet every day to reap the gut-health benefits.

Fermented foods – Fermented foods are gut-friendly thanks to the good bacteria (probiotics) they contain, but they are not something we typically eat much of in this country. They are now appearing on the supermarket shelves, so give them a go:

- Kefir is a fermented milk product, rather like sour yogurt. It's good in smoothies, or you can include it in your overnight oats (see Ten-plant-foods Overnight Oats on page 179).

- Kimchi is a Korean dish of spicy fermented cabbage. It's usually served as a condiment, but also pairs well with eggs (see Kimchi and Spring Onion Omelette on page 184) or cheese.

- Kombucha is a fermented tea product that is a great alternative to an alcoholic aperitif.

- Tempeh is a fermented soy bean product that comes in a block that you can cut up into pieces and use as a meat replacement

Gut health recap

- A healthy gut is one that has a diverse range of good bacteria, and is resilient and stable.
- A healthy gut supports overall health, but in particular weight management, brain health and immunity.
- The single best way to support your gut health is to eat 30 different plant foods a week. This includes all fruit and vegetables, grains and legumes, nuts and seeds, and herbs and spices.
- A healthy, balanced, inclusive diet is best for gut health. Do not cut out foods or food groups unless you have a condition that requires you to do so.
- Cleanses and detoxes do not support gut health, and in some cases may be detrimental to gut bacteria diversity.
- The efficacy of probiotic supplements is unclear. Eating a gut-friendly diet is the best way to support gut health.
- If you experience gut-health issues, see a doctor to get a proper diagnosis. Some conditions, like coeliac disease, can be tested for, and there are dietary interventions like the FODMAP diet that can be helpful with conditions like IBS when done under supervision.
- Eating fermented, probiotic and prebiotic foods is a good way to improve your gut health.

in stir-fries and curries (see Indonesian Vegetables and Tempeh in a Coconut Milk Broth on page 188).

- Other more familiar fermented foods include sauerkraut and miso paste.

Other probiotic foods – If you really can't get to grips with fermented foods, there are other options that contain those good bacteria but without the funky tang. Live yogurt and cheese with live cultures, including Parmesan, feta, Edam, Gouda, Emmental, mozzarella, unpasteurised Cheddar and cottage cheese, are all good options.

Prebiotic foods – To recap, prebiotic foods contain resistant starch, which ferments in the gut to feed the good bacteria. Prebiotic foods include bananas, leeks, garlic, onions, asparagus, barley, oats and cooked and cooled rice.

Ten easy ways to support your gut health

1. **Sign-up to a box scheme** – Joining a local fruit and veg box scheme means a regular delivery of varied produce. There will be things in there you don't usually buy, so you will be expanding your plant-food consumption every week.

2. **Add more herbs and spices to meals** – Herbs can be added to salads and sprinkled over most meals. Sweet spices, like cinnamon, nutmeg and allspice, can be added to smoothies, porridge and pancake mixes. Add extra savoury spices to dishes you already make; for example, try adding cumin to scrambled eggs, turmeric to salad dressings, etc.

3. **Eat seeds and nuts every day** – They are excellent as a snack, but can also be added to your favourite dishes. Toast some to add crunch to soups and salads in place of croutons. Nut butters are also a convenient way to eat more nuts. Try the Nut Butter-stuffed Frozen Dates on page 240.

4. **Throw in a tin.** You'll see this advice given often throughout this book. Get into the habit of adding a tin of beans or lentils to curries, soups or stews, or make them the main event, like in the tasty Creamy Bean and Mushroom Stew on page 172.

5. **Stock up on pre-cooked pouches.** Again, you will see this advice repeated in several chapters of this book, as it is an easy way to tick lots of nutritional boxes. A pouch of pre-cooked mixed grains is used in the Good Guts Prebiotic Soup on page 180.

6. **Don't forget frozen.** Frozen fruits and vegetables can be used in smoothies, and good old-fashioned frozen peas and sweetcorn all count. Frozen spinach works well in curries.

7. **Mix it up.** Opt for a bag of mixed salad rather than a one-leaf variety. Go for different colours of the same veg, e.g. red, yellow and green peppers, red and white onions and cabbage. Buy packets of mixed seeds and nuts. Buy tins and pouches of mixed beans and grains.

8. **Include at least two plant foods at every single meal.** For example, swap out your Marmite on toast for avocado and tomato on toast, or top your oats with mixed berries and mixed seeds.

9. **Ditch processed snacks.** Switch to gut-friendly snacks like wholegrain rice cakes and crackers, nuts, fruit or hummus and veggie sticks.

10. **Eat a 'K food' every day.** Keep some kimchi, kefir, kombucha or kraut in the fridge and have some every day. You can even try making your own Easy Kimchi (see page 182). If you really don't like fermented foods, live yogurt is a good alternative.

SIX

Get Your Five-a-day

Why is it important to have plenty of fruit and vegetables in the diet?

This may seem like a really silly question, because we all know fruit and vegetables are good for us. They provide all sorts of vitamins and minerals, the antioxidant polyphenols they contain give them their vibrant colour, and they are a source of healthy complex carbs and fibre. But research is now exploring beyond the traditional findings that fruit and vegetables can reduce the risk of cancer and heart attacks, and looking at the psychological benefits too.

A 2021 study found that eating a diet rich in fruit and vegetables was associated with less stress. The findings revealed that people who ate at least 470g of fruit and vegetables daily had 10% lower stress levels than those who consumed less than 230g.[46]

And it's not just helpful for stress; research from the University of Warwick found that eating more fruit and vegetables can substantially increase people's happiness levels. The researchers concluded that people who changed from almost no fruit and veg to eight portions of fruit and veg a day experienced an increase in life satisfaction equivalent to moving from unemployment to employment.[47]

It's clear that eating plenty of fruit and vegetables is a no-brainer – there isn't a dietitian in the world who doesn't agree with that – but what is less clear is *how much* we should be eating.

Why is it five-a-day? I've heard it should be eight or even ten-a-day.

The first thing to say here is that any fruit and vegetables are better than nothing, so even if the idea of five portions a day seems a lot, the first step is simply to make sure you are eating some every day and vary what you have as much as possible.

There have been numerous reports over the years suggesting that five-a-day isn't sufficient for good health, and we should be aiming for more. One 2017 study by University College London concluded that ten-a-day should be the target – surely a tall order for even the most eager veggie-botherer.

But more recently, a comprehensive 2021 review by the American Heart Association of studies representing nearly 2 million adults worldwide found that eating five daily servings of fruits and vegetables (of which two were fruit and three were vegetables) was the optimal amount for a longer life.[48] Eating more than five servings was not associated with any additional health benefits.

So, for now, we stick with five portions of fruit and veg a day, a realistic and achievable target for most of us, but of course there's nothing to stop you eating more than this if you wish to. But what constitutes a 'portion' of fruit or vegetables? According to current NHS guidelines, it's as follows:[49]

- 80g of fresh, tinned or frozen fruit and vegetables

- 30g of dried fruit

Note that the following only count once a day:

- 150ml of fruit juice, vegetable juice or smoothies. This is limited to a combined total of 150ml a day because of the high sugar content.

- 80g of beans and pulses. These only count once as part of your five-a-day even if you eat more than that, because although they're a good source of fibre, they contain fewer nutrients than other fruits and vegetables.

But 80g can be hard to visualise; any idea what 80g of strawberries looks like, anyone? It might be worth weighing your fruit and vegetables for a time, or looking at the weights given on the packets you buy, just to get an idea of what 80g looks like for each kind. For a more detailed breakdown, see Appendix A (pages 255–7), which gives the NHS portion-size guidelines in full.

But isn't fruit full of sugar?

Fruits contain varying amounts of sugar in the form of fructose. There has been much debate about how fructose should be regarded in terms of sugar in the diet. If we are trying to reduce sugar overall, surely we need to reduce our fruit consumption?

The point here is that fruit generally has a low GI; as you will remember, we talked about glycaemic index and glycaemic load in the carbs chapter (see page 28). Because fruit is a whole food, you are getting a package of nutrition: yes, this includes fructose, but also plenty of fibre, so the energy is released slowly and doesn't cause blood sugar spikes. Fruits are also packed with micronutrients and other helpful compounds like polyphenols which are all beneficial to health. So as far as fruit is concerned, you don't need to be overly concerned about the sugar content.

The only caveat to this is if you are juicing your fruit, because this will remove most of the fibre and effectively produce a liquid of concentrated fructose. This is why you should have no more than 150ml of juice per day. Shop-bought smoothies, similarly, can be very high in sugar, but the ones you make at home are better because you can control their contents to include grains, nuts and vegetables as well as fruit, creating a more nutritious and balanced blend. The smoothie recipes in this book are designed to be beneficial in this way.

What's the best way to make sure I eat my five-a-day?

If we are aiming for a minimum of five portions of fruit and vegetables a day, you need to include two at each meal or have one at each meal and two snacks comprising one portion each.

You may have heard the phrase 'eat the rainbow'. This is not only a great rule for creating visually appetising meals; colour is also nature's way of signalling the health benefits of a particular plant. Try to eat a range of fruit and vegetables across these colour groupings:

Blue and purple – Blue and purple fruit and vegetables are extremely high in antioxidant anthocyanins, which research has linked to a wide variety of health benefits, including increased longevity, cardiovascular health, cancer prevention and reduced risk of cognitive decline and dementia. Choose from:

> blackberries
> blueberries
> black cherries
> black plums
> figs
> aubergines
> red onions
> purple sprouting broccoli
> beetroot
> red cabbage

Green – Green fruit and vegetables contain glucosinolates, lutein, zeaxanthin and folic acid, all of which are known to reduce the risk of cancer. Choose from:

> green apples
> green grapes
> limes
> kiwi fruit

pears
spinach and other leafy greens like kale
green herbs
celery
cucumbers
broccoli
sprouts
pak choy
asparagus
courgettes
green beans
green cabbage
green peppers
peas
avocados
green chillies

Orange – Orange fruit and vegetables are high in carotenoids, crucial for supporting your immune system, cell repair and good vision. Choose from:

oranges
tangerines
apricots
nectarines
peaches
papayas
mangoes
passion fruit
cantaloupe melons
carrots
pumpkins
squash
sweet potatoes
orange peppers
turmeric

Yellow – Yellow fruit and vegetables contain large amounts of bioflavonoids, which help reduce inflammation and fight infection. Choose from:

> pineapples
> lemons
> golden kiwis
> yellow watermelons
> bananas
> ginger
> sweetcorn
> yellow peppers
> yellow tomatoes
> yellow courgettes

Red – Red fruit and vegetables contain plant chemicals including lycopene, ellagic acid and a flavonoid called kaempferol. These can be cancer protective and can also help reduce the risk of heart disease. Choose from:

> red cherries
> red apples
> strawberries
> raspberries
> red grapes
> pink grapefruit
> rhubarb
> watermelons
> cranberries
> pomegranates
> tomatoes
> red peppers
> radicchio
> radishes
> red chillies

Five-a-day recap

- Fruit and vegetables contain important micronutrients and fibre, which are crucial for all aspects of our physical and mental health.
- Current research still supports the guidance to eat five portions of fruit and vegetables a day. A portion is 80g.
- The sugar contained in whole fruit comes as a complete nutritional package, including fibre, so we don't need to be concerned about it in the same way that we are with 'free' sugars, which spike blood sugar levels.
- Remember to 'eat the rainbow'. Choose fruit and vegetables of different colours to ensure you are getting a range of phytochemicals, vitamins and minerals for maximum health benefits.

Ten easy ways to get your five-a-day

1. **Start with a smoothie.** Breakfast smoothies are a nutritious way to start the day, but remember this only counts as one of your five-a-day. Try the Sunshine Smoothie on page 190.

2. **Add vegetables and herbs to your morning eggs.** Tomatoes, avocados, spring onions, mushrooms, parsley, basil and chives are all good options. For a fabulous brunch idea, try the Rainbow Vegetable Crustless Quiche on page 219.

3. **Get a Sunday soup habit.** Make a veggie-packed soup on a Sunday to have for lunches in the week. Try the delicious Many Veg and Cheddar Soup on page 191.

4. **Remember the half-plate rule.** At mealtimes, fill half your plate with a selection of vegetables/salad. Balance with complex carbs and lean protein (see previous chapters for guidance on portion size for these macronutrients).

5. **Go raw.** Raw slaw is another easy way to up your veg intake with a simple, healthy side dish. One of my favourite versions is Curtido (Mexican Slaw) on page 193.

6. **Herbs are not just a garnish!** Use herbs in salads in quantity – you can add large handfuls of chopped parsley, basil or mint to most salads, or even all three.

7. **Vary the veg.** Rather than have a single vegetable as a side dish, eat more by mixing two or three. See page 200 for my Garlic Greens recipe, which is the perfect accompaniment to any meat or fish dish.

8. **Roast some veggies.** Roasting vegetables like onions, sweet potatoes, butternut squash, tomatoes and courgettes together is a great way to eat a wider variety, and it also intensifies their flavours. My Roasted Roots with Feta and Mint on page 128 is a delicious example.

9. **Bring back the side salad.** Side salads seem a bit retro these days, but if you have a selection of stuff from the salad drawer on the table at dinnertime alongside whatever else you are eating, you'll clock up a couple of extra portions of veg each day.

10. **Snack on fruits and vegetables.** If you focus on eating fruit and vegetables at snack time, it will be far easier to reach your five-a-day target. See pages 99–100 for some healthy snack ideas.

SEVEN

Get Your Vitamins and Minerals In

What are vitamins and minerals, and why does my body need them?

As children, we were told to eat our greens, as if vegetables were the only foods containing any goodness. Thankfully, vitamins and minerals are found in a wide range of plant foods, as well as in meat, fish, dairy and eggs.

Vitamins and minerals, otherwise known as micronutrients, are simply compounds required by the body in very small amounts for a variety of essential processes, including keeping our bones, muscles, hearts and brains working properly.

Most micronutrients cannot be made by the body, and so need to come from our diets. The exception is vitamin D, which can be made in the skin when we are exposed to sunlight. Vitamins are grouped into fat-soluble vitamins (A, D, E and K) and water-soluble vitamins (all the B vitamins and C). Minerals we need to include in our diet include calcium, copper, iodine, iron, magnesium, manganese, phosphorus, potassium, selenium and zinc. Sodium and chloride are also important minerals, but as these are found in salt, which is widely consumed, we are unlikely to be deficient.

I've heard that the foods we eat these days aren't as rich in vitamins and minerals as they used to be.

There has been much written about the mineral nutrient composition of vegetables, fruits and grains declining over the past 50 years, but a comprehensive 2017 study review came to the following conclusions:[50]

- The mineral nutrient composition of vegetables, fruits and grains is not declining.

- Allegations of decline due to agricultural soil mineral depletion are unfounded.

- Some high-yield varieties show a dilution effect of lower mineral concentrations.

- Changes are within natural variation ranges and are not nutritionally significant.

- Eating the recommended daily servings provides adequate nutrition.

Are there any circumstances in which a multivitamin and mineral supplement might be advisable?

The focus of this book is to empower you to get everything you need nutritionally from your food. I call it a 'food first' approach. Having said that, there are some instances where targeted supplementation may be advisable, as discussed on pages 16–19.

In truth, there is little harm in taking a good-quality multivitamin and mineral supplement if you feel reassured by doing so, but you should also know that the health benefits of taking them remain largely unproven. The case for supplementation is certainly stronger if you are on a restricted diet for any reason, or if you have a medical condition that makes it harder to absorb what you need from your food.

It is important to remember that a pill is no substitute for a healthy, well-balanced diet. If you are popping supplements because you feel it lets you off the hook nutritionally, then you may be doing more harm than good. At the end of the day, the body is designed to digest food, not pills, and supplements don't contain the other nutritional goodies found in real food, like healthy fats, fibre and health-giving phytochemicals.

Which foods contain which micronutrients and how much of them do I need?

In the UK, we have a system called the Reference Nutrient Intake, or RNI, which specifies a recommended daily amount for each nutrient. For example, it's advised that we have 40mg of vitamin C per day. In my experience, it's not a very helpful system, because in all honesty, who can be bothered to calculate what quantity of each food source of vitamin C delivers the requisite dose, and eat accordingly?

The picture is further complicated when you consider the role of bioavailability – or how easily micronutrients are absorbed by the body. Bioavailability of the micronutrients in our food is affected by a whole host of factors, such as gender, age, our own nutrient store of a particular nutrient, how food is cooked and processed and, in some cases, interactions between different foods. In summary, it's virtually impossible to calculate how much of any particular micronutrient we are absorbing. You can see why it's so tempting for people to resort to supplements as a kind of insurance policy.

The truth is that we don't really need to worry about daily intakes per se, as you are unlikely to be deficient in any of the key micronutrients if you have a basic understanding of which foods contain them and you eat a wide range of these foods over the course of a week. Here's a quick guide to the main food sources for the key micronutrients. There are, of course, lots of others, but if you are regularly eating foods from the following list, you are going to be covering your bases – and if not, it will help you to plug the gaps.

Micronutrient	Main Food Sources[51]
Vitamin A	Tuna, carrots, butternut squash, sweet potatoes, red peppers, spinach, lettuce, broccoli, cantaloupe melons, pink grapefruit.
Vitamin B1 (thiamin)	Pork, salmon, shellfish, soy, squash, asparagus, peas, black beans, brown rice, flaxseeds.
Vitamin B2 (riboflavin)	Beef, pork, fish, milk, eggs, soy, mushrooms, spinach, avocados, almonds.
Vitamin B3 (niacin)	Beef, pork, chicken, fish, avocados, mushrooms, green peas, sweet potatoes, brown rice, peanuts.
Vitamin B5 (pantothenic acid)	Beef, pork, chicken, trout, milk, avocados, mushrooms, sweet potatoes, lentils, sunflower seeds.
Vitamin B6 (pyridoxine)	Beef, pork, chicken, salmon, tofu or tempeh, avocados, potatoes, sweet potatoes, bananas, pistachios.
Vitamin B7 (biotin)	Liver, eggs, avocados, broccoli, mushrooms, sweet potatoes, bananas, legumes, nuts, seeds.
Vitamin B9 (folate/folic acid)	Edamame beans, avocados, asparagus, lettuce, sweetcorn, spinach, broccoli, mangoes, lentils, wholegrain bread.
Vitamin B12 (cobalamin)	Beef, oily fish, shellfish, fortified vegan products like tofu and non-dairy milks, milk, cheese, eggs, yeast extract spreads, almonds.
Vitamin C	Broccoli, mangetout, kale, tomatoes, peppers, guavas, kiwi fruit, strawberries, oranges, papayas.
Vitamin D	Oily fish, mushrooms, pork, eggs, dairy products fortified with vitamin D.
Vitamin E	Trout, prawns, spinach, avocados, butternut squash, kiwi fruit, olive oil, almonds, sunflower seeds.

Ten Easy Ways to Get Everything You Need from Your Food

Micronutrient	Main Food Sources
Vitamin K	Kale, broccoli, Brussels sprouts, cabbage, fennel, broad beans, green beans, asparagus, kiwi fruit, salad leaves.
Calcium	Tinned fish including the bones (like sardines), tofu or tempeh, milk, yogurt, cheese, broccoli, kale, white beans, almonds, sesame seeds.
Copper	Salmon, shellfish, tofu or tempeh, avocados, mushrooms, sweet potatoes, chickpeas, cashews, sesame seeds, dark chocolate.
Iodine	Sea fish (cod, sardines, salmon, tuna), shellfish, prawns, seaweed and other sea vegetables, dairy, eggs, prunes, butter beans, iodised salt.
Iron	Beef, shellfish, dark leafy greens, mushrooms, dried fruit, beans, lentils, quinoa, pumpkin seeds, dark chocolate.
Magnesium	Tuna, plain yogurt, avocados, spinach, bananas, butter beans, brown rice, almonds, pumpkin seeds, dark chocolate.
Manganese	Shellfish, soy, spinach, sweet potatoes, pineapples, white beans, chickpeas, oats, brown rice, almonds.
Phosphorus	Beef, pork, chicken, oily fish, shellfish, milk, butternut squash, lentils, oats, quinoa, pumpkin seeds.
Potassium	Salmon, milk, leafy green vegetables, avocados, potatoes, pumpkin and squash, mushrooms, cooked tomatoes, bananas, white beans.
Selenium	Beef, pork, chicken, tuna, prawns and shellfish, tofu or tempeh, mushrooms, wholemeal pasta, Brazil nuts.
Zinc	Beef, chicken, pork, oysters, tofu, yogurt, mushrooms, lentils, oats, seeds.

Vitamins and minerals recap

- Vitamins and minerals, otherwise known as micronutrients, are compounds required in small amounts for many essential processes in the body.
- Most need to come from what we eat, with the exception of vitamin D, which our body makes in the skin upon exposure to the sun.
- Rather than focusing on the RNI for each micronutrient, eating a wide range of foods containing the essential vitamins and minerals over the course of a week is the best way to ensure you are getting what you require.
- The bioavailability of micronutrients is important, and there are a few simple things you can do to maximise the absorption of key vitamins and minerals that we will cover below.

Ten easy ways to maximise your micronutrients

1. **Eat a wide variety of foods.** The best overall advice for maximising micronutrient intake is to eat a combination of fruit and vegetables, wholegrain carbohydrates, lean protein and healthy fat at every meal, as different food groups provide different nutrients.

2. **Eat locally grown fruit and vegetables.** It's estimated that by the time you buy produce at the supermarket, it can have lost up to half of its vitamin and mineral content, depending on how long ago it was picked. Signing up to a local box scheme or buying from a local greengrocer are good ways to ensure the fruit and veg you eat are as fresh as possible.

3. Cut them up. Cutting up fruits and vegetables before eating releases the nutrients by helping to break down the cell walls. For example, crushing garlic releases a compound called allicin, which can help lower cholesterol and blood pressure levels.

4. Store your fresh produce properly. This will slow down nutrient loss:

- Store all vegetables, except root vegetables, in the refrigerator.

- Store all fruits except berries (this includes tomatoes and avocados) at room temperature away from direct light.

- Cover cut fruits and vegetables with a squeeze of lemon juice to prevent oxidation and store in an airtight container in the fridge.

5. Be careful with cooking. Some micronutrients are water-soluble and sensitive to heat, especially the B vitamins and vitamin C. Cooking foods containing these vitamins in water can reduce their nutrient content (see box below for tips on how to retain more nutrients when cooking). A good idea is to use them in soups so that any vitamins that have leached out are still consumed (see the Many Veg and Cheddar Soup on page 191).

6. But cooking can be good. In some instances, cooking can actually *increase* the level of certain nutrients. For example, lycopene increases by 25% when tomatoes are cooked, and the bioavailability of beta-carotene – found in red, orange and yellow plants like tomatoes, peppers, carrots and sweet potatoes – is also increased by cooking. Try the Roasted Veg Greek Salad on page 194.

7. Absorb more of the nutrients you eat. The bioavailability of certain nutrients is aided by pairing with other foods. For example, foods containing the fat-soluble vitamins A, D, E and K should be eaten with some healthy fats like nuts, avocado or olive oil. To better absorb the iron from foods, pair with vitamin C from sources such as berries, citrus fruit, tomatoes and peppers, for example the Nutrify Salad on page 210.

8. **Vitamin D is key for calcium.** Vitamin D is required to enhance the absorption of calcium, so consume vitamin D-rich foods with calcium-rich foods. Try the Hot-smoked Salmon Smash-up (page 241), which pairs oily fish for vitamin D with calcium from Greek yogurt.

9. **Animal sources are better for some micronutrients.** If you are not vegan or vegetarian, the animal-based sources of some

Cooking some foods can reduce their nutrient content. Here are some simple tips to minimise nutrient loss:

- Cook vegetables in smaller amounts of water to reduce the loss of vitamins B and C. You can keep any liquid left in the pan to use in soups and stews, or use it to make up stock cubes.
- Cook vegetables lightly; steaming, quick stir-frying and blanching for a few minutes are better than boiling.
- Don't peel vegetables, as fewer nutrients will be lost if the skins are kept on.
- Try to eat any cooked vegetables within a day or two, as their vitamin C content will continue to reduce with exposure to the air.
- Cut up food after cooking rather than before, as that way less of it will have been directly exposed to heat and water.
- When cooking meat, poultry and fish, use the shortest cooking time needed for safe consumption.
- Pour any juices that escape from resting meat back over it before eating.

key vitamins and minerals are usually more bioavailable than plant-based sources. This is especially true for vitamins A and B, as well as iron, calcium, magnesium and zinc. For this reason, animal-based sources are well represented in the recipe section of this book, such as the Simple Lamb and Chickpea Tagine on page 216.

10. **Don't forget frozen.** When fruit and vegetables are out of season, buy them frozen – they are cheaper, and also more likely to retain the micronutrients they contained when picked. For example, the Healthy Palak Paneer (page 214) uses frozen spinach.

EIGHT

Keep an Eye on Calories

What are calories and why does my body need them?

Calories have become a loaded term, and even nutritionists are divided. Some think it's important to calorie-count in order to manage our weight, while others feel it's a reductionist approach that is outdated and unhelpful.

Wherever you sit on the question of calories, it's important to understand that they are simply a measurement of the amount of energy contained within food. This energy is processed a little differently from person to person according to our unique physiologies, and different foods have different thermic effects (the thermic effect is the amount of energy it takes for your body to digest, absorb, and metabolise the food). But the fact remains that if you consume more energy than you expend, you will end up putting on weight.

Although this book is about supercharging your diet and not about weight management, it is important to have one eye on your energy intake, because even a diet containing lots of nutritious foods can end up being overly calorific. The health impacts of being overweight and obese are well documented, from an increased risk of cancer to cardiovascular disease and type 2 diabetes.

What is a healthy weight?

A healthy weight is one that falls within a weight range that is not associated with an increased risk of disease and ill-health. The NHS base their calculation of what constitutes a healthy weight on Body Mass Index (BMI), a formula that divides a person's weight by the square of their height. Adults with a BMI of 18.5 to 24.9 are considered to be a healthy weight; those with a BMI of 25 to 29.9 are considered to be overweight; and those with a BMI of over 30 are considered to be obese.[52]

While BMI can be a useful indicator, it is not reliable when applied to certain demographics. For example, elderly adults who may have lost some muscle and bone mass could have a BMI in the normal range, but might actually be carrying too much body fat. Similarly, people with a high muscle-to-fat ratio might have a higher BMI because muscle weighs more than fat.

Recent guidelines from NICE (the National Institute for Health and Care Excellence) advise that our waist circumference is a better indicator of whether or not we are a healthy weight, and aiming to keep your waist measurement to less than half your height reduces the risk of potential health problems.[53] So, a person who is 170cm tall should have a waist circumference of 85cm or less.

How many calories do I need?

The blanket guideline for calorie needs as published on the NHS website is 2,500 per day for an adult man and 2,000 per day for an adult woman. Clearly, this is far too blunt an instrument to be helpful when trying to manage our weight, as it doesn't consider factors such as age or lifestyle. The right amount of calories is effectively the amount of calories you can eat at any point in time without putting on weight. For most of us, it's a case of trial and error, but there are calorie calculators online that will help you arrive at a rough figure for your likely daily calorie requirement.

Don't count calories, make calories count

Figuring out your daily calorie allowance is one thing, but unless you are counting calories, how much use is it to you? For most of us, calorie-counting – or tracking, as it's more often called nowadays –

is impractical and not something we want to do day in, day out. It can also lead us to focus too much on calories to the detriment of considering the nutritional value of our food.

However, we do need to be somewhat mindful of the energy content of the foods we are consuming so we can manage our weight. I prefer to think of it as being 'calorie-aware' rather than calorie-counting; in other words, having a sense of the relative calorie loads of different foods rather than knowing the exact calorie count.

And being calorie-aware doesn't just apply to those foods we know are not so good for us; even some healthy things are surprisingly calorific. Foods like avocados, nuts and nut butters, granola, energy balls and vegan desserts incorporating lots of nuts, seeds and oil are very high in calories, so portion control is key.

Given we only have a certain amount of calories to play with, we need to make those calories count. I call this your 'food spend'. Think of your calories as a currency; you've only got a fixed amount to spend in a day, so be judicious about your purchases.

Something that can be helpful in this regard is the Aggregate Nutrient Density Index (ANDI), which ranks the nutrient value of many foods on the basis of how many micronutrients they deliver to your body for each calorie consumed. They are ranked on a scale of 1–1,000 with 1,000 being the most nutrient-dense. See Appendix B (page 258) for a sample listing of common foods and their ANDI scores.

This information can be helpful if you are trying to lose weight healthily because you can see which foods are nutritious but lower in calories. But a word of caution: the ANDI takes no account of macronutrient balance in the diet. Clearly a diet consisting of only leafy greens, which appear at the top of the list, would not be a healthy one. Some healthy foods, like avocados, can rank quite low on the scale, simply because they are higher in calories.

The recipes in the Lower-calorie Meals section later on (pages 218–32) have been designed to incorporate nutrient-dense foods while still maintaining a good macro balance.

Calories recap

- Calories are simply a measure of the energy content of food. Energy is required by the body to function.
- If we consume more energy than we expend, we will put on weight; it's for this reason we have to keep an eye on our calorie intake.
- A healthy weight varies from person to person, but the latest advice is to try and keep your waist measurement to under half your height.
- Our daily calorie requirement also varies from person to person depending on various factors. You can use an online calorie calculator to get an idea of what yours might be.
- You don't need to count calories in order to be calorie-aware. Understanding the rough calorie loads of different foods will enable you to manage your weight more effectively.
- When in weight-loss mode, it can be helpful to focus on foods that are lower in calories but very nutrient-dense, but remember you still need to eat a healthy, balanced diet overall.

Ten easy ways to keep an eye on calories

1. Practise calorie-shaving. For example:

- Instead of milky coffees like lattes, stick to black coffee with a splash of milk and don't add sugar.

- Ditch processed sauces like mayonnaise and tomato ketchup; these add calories (and often free sugars) to your meal.

- Make your own homemade salad dressings rather than using shop-bought ones, and use them sparingly.

- Make lower-calorie substitutions. For example, if a recipe calls for soured cream or mayonnaise, use Greek yogurt instead.

2. Stick to water. Don't drink your calories, as they all add up.

3. Watch your portion sizes. Keep an eye on your portion sizes, as some healthy foods are high in calories:

- nut butter – 100 calories per tablespoon

- tahini – 100 calories per tablespoon

- nuts, seeds, granola – 180 calories per 30g

- olive oil – 120 calories per tablespoon

- coconut milk – 230 calories per 100ml (use a light version, which has 115 calories per 100ml)

- avocados – 80 calories per ¼ avocado

- oily fish, e.g. salmon – 210 calories per 100g

- dried fruit – raisins (90 calories per 30g); dried apricots (60 calories per 30g)

- bread – 100 calories per regular slice

4. Focus on healthy foods that are lower in calories. Eat plenty of these foods, which deliver good nutrition with a lower food spend:

- Greek yogurt – the Smoked Mackerel Pâté on Toast with Watercress and an Egg (page 225) uses Greek yogurt in place of the usual cream cheese.

- Eggs – the Rainbow Vegetable Crustless Quiche (page 219) has all the goodness of eggs and veggies without the calorific pastry.

- White fish – hake is a sustainable and lower-calorie choice of fish; try the delicious Hake Pomodoro with White Beans on page 231.

- Beans, lentils and chickpeas – try the Roast Chicken with Herby Harissa Puy Lentils (page 229) for a fabulous way to incorporate lentils in a lower-calorie dish.

- Oats, quinoa and brown rice – the Raspberry Ripple Porridge (page 218) is an ideal way to start the day, with wholegrains and fibre-rich raspberries.

- All fruit, but especially berries, melons, papaya, apples and grapefruit.

- All vegetables and salad. Try the Spinach, Squash and Red Onion Salad with Halloumi Croutons and a Sweet Chilli Dressing (page 223).

- Fresh herbs and spices, lemon juice and vinegars add flavour to meals – the Spaghetti with Peas, Asparagus and Hot-smoked Salmon (page 227) uses lemon and dill to good effect.

5. **Use the 20% rule.** Think about the overall quantity of food on your plate. Try taking 20% less than you usually do, and only have more if you are genuinely still hungry.

6. **Include some protein with every meal.** This will help satiety and you will be less likely to overeat.

7. **Fibre, fibre, fibre.** Make sure to eat plenty of fibre, as this will keep you feeling full for longer, and it helps you digest the food

you are eating more efficiently. Revisit the fibre section (pages 55–62) for tips on how to do this.

8. **Eat slowly and without distractions.** By allowing your gut to catch up with your mouth, you will feel more satisfied with a smaller volume of food.

9. **Avoid desserts.** If you feel the need for something sweet at the end of your evening meal, have a square or two of dark chocolate (at least 85% cocoa solids).

10. **Don't snack after dinner.** Eating after dinner is a common way to overshoot on calories. If you are a night-time snacker, the next section, 'Snack Smart', will help you break the habit.

NINE

Snack Smart

Is snacking good or bad for you?

You'd be forgiven for asking this question, but in truth it's one that neatly sums up our dysfunctional relationship with food. Attaching a moral value to what we eat is something we need to move away from. Instead of thinking about food in terms of 'good' or 'bad', what we should ask ourselves instead is: is snacking beneficial for my body?

The answer to this question is, it depends. We are all different. Some of us might describe ourselves as grazers, needing regular energy boosts throughout the day; others might breeze from meal to meal without so much as a glance at the fridge.

According to a recent study by King's College London, the explanation for this may partly lie in how your blood sugar levels respond to meals. Participants experiencing a more pronounced blood sugar dip after eating a meal (referred to as 'big dippers') were far more likely to have cravings and, subsequently, to snack.[54]

And then there are lifestyle factors to consider. If you have a physical job or do lots of exercise, then snacking can be a genuine response to your body's needs. The NHS Guidelines on Food and Drink for Sport advise that having a light snack that contains some protein and is higher in carbohydrates and lower in fat can help you perform during your training and recover afterwards.

While our physiology and lifestyles certainly account for some of our propensity to graze, we often head to the kitchen for reasons that have little to do with hunger. Who hasn't found themselves nose-deep in a packet of crisps when bored, stressed or perhaps just needing a break from work?

In summary, snacking is fine as long as it is in response to a genuine nutritional need – and, of course, it depends on what you choose to snack on.

To snack or not to snack?

The first step when it comes to deciding whether or not to have a snack is to identify your trigger times for snacking. Here are some common ones:

- following exercise

- mid-morning, if you haven't had a balanced breakfast

- late afternoon, when you may experience low blood sugar

- habitual snacking after dinner, perhaps in front of the TV

When you get the urge to snack, the key is to pause and assess the situation by asking yourself these questions:

1. How hungry am I, on a scale of one to ten?

2. Am I just bored, or am I using snacking as a way to take a break?

3. Might I be thirsty? Thirst and hunger are often confused.

If you assess your hunger as anything below a seven, you don't really need a snack, particularly if it's not too long until your next meal. If you are just bored or needing a break, then distraction is the best strategy, so do something else instead that doesn't involve eating. Take a short walk and listen to a podcast; if it's later in the day, have a bath or shower, or roll out a mat and do a ten-minute yoga session.

If you decide you are hungry and do want a snack, first have a glass of water to rule out the possibility that you are simply dehydrated. Wait a few minutes and see if that does the trick. If not, then have something to eat, but what you choose to snack on is key when it comes to supercharging your diet.

What should I snack on, and what's the appropriate portion size?

When you snack, ideally you want it to contribute to your nutritional goals for the day. So far in this book, we've covered the importance of complex carbs, lean protein, healthy fats and getting enough fibre. We've also discussed foods that are good for gut health, getting enough fruit and vegetables, making sure all our micronutrients are covered, and making sure we don't blow our daily calorie allowance.

By choosing the right *kind* of snack, you can help tick many of those nutritional boxes. Here are some tasty, healthy snacks that won't break the calorie bank:

1 medium pear and 20g pistachios – Provides one of your five-a-day and plenty of fibre. The nuts also contain healthy fat and plant protein to fill you up.

1 apple and 20g almonds – Apples contain pectin, a prebiotic that's good for gut health, and the almonds are packed with vitamin E.

50g berries and 2 tablespoons Greek yogurt – Berries are low in sugar and high in antioxidants. The protein in the yogurt will improve appetite control, so you are less likely to overeat at your next meal.

1 small banana and 20g peanuts – A great flavour combination as well as providing fibre, fat and protein.

Some carrot sticks with 1 tablespoon hummus – The crunchy texture of the carrots is satisfying, and they are sweet without being high in sugar. Pair with hummus for a balanced, satisfying snack.

1 celery stick with 1 tablespoon nut butter – Celery is refreshing and hydrating, and the nut butter provides complex carbs, healthy fat and plant protein, balancing up the macronutrients nicely.

Snack smart recap

- Snacking is fine if it is in response to genuine hunger.
- Learn to tune into your snacking triggers, and assess your hunger level.
- If you don't really need a snack try and distract yourself with another activity.
- If you do need something to eat choose a snack that is nutritious and filling.

1 wholegrain cracker with 1 tablespoon cream cheese – This is a good snack if you fancy something savoury and crunchy in place of crisps. Choose a wholegrain cracker for more plant-food goodness; you could even try making your own Super Seedy Crackers (page 244). The cream cheese ticks the protein and fat boxes for satiety.

A square of dark chocolate (at least 85% cocoa solids) and a few salted peanuts – A healthy Snickers bar, if you will. Polyphenols in the dark chocolate are heart-healthy and the peanuts are rich in protein, fat and fibre.

Ten easy ways to snack smart

1. **Drink first.** Remember the tip to have a glass of water first if you feel hungry and see if the feeling passes.

2. **Think 'nutrients first' when it comes to snacks.** If you still want a snack, think about what it delivers nutritionally. Is it balanced (carbs, fat, protein)? Does it provide some vitamins and minerals? Remember, that snack can either help or hinder your healthy-eating goals.

3. **Take time to eat your snack.** Once you've chosen your snack, eat it slowly and chew it thoroughly, especially nuts. One study found that people who chewed almonds thoroughly (up to 40 chews) felt full longer than those who chewed the same amount of nuts fewer times.[55]

4. **Pack a snack.** Have snacks with you when out and about or at work, so that you don't end up resorting to something unhealthy. Fruit is easy to pack, or you could make some of my fibre-rich Prune Power Balls (page 238).

5. **Develop snack strategies.** Identify your weaknesses (e.g. biscuits), assess when you usually eat them and why (e.g. late-afternoon energy lull), and develop a strategy (e.g. switch to a healthier snack at that time instead – see below).

6. **Make your own healthy sweet snacks.** We all crave something sweet from time to time. Make your own healthy Nut Butter-stuffed Frozen Dates (page 240) to have instead of a biscuit.

7. **Out of sight, out of mind.** If you live alone, an easy solution is not to have unhealthy snack foods in the house. If you live with others, this isn't so easy, but just make sure snack foods are stored out of sight and are not easily accessible, so you aren't tempted to grab something every time you go into the kitchen. And don't keep snacks in the car!

8. **Mealtimes matter.** Don't go too long between meals; if you don't space out your meals evenly throughout the day, you will inevitably end up ravenous and susceptible to random snacking.

9. **Nix the night-time snacks.** Ideally, you don't want to eat within a couple of hours of bedtime, but equally don't have dinner too early or you'll be hungry again before bed. An evening meal with a good macronutrient balance is more likely to stabilise your blood sugar levels and reduce cravings.

10. **Try a tea.** If you still feel like a late-night snack, try having a drink that promotes good sleep instead, such as chamomile, peppermint or valerian tea – or make the Sleeping Potion on page 253.

TEN

Think About What You Drink

Why do we need to think about what we drink?

It's easy to ignore drinks when it comes to nutrition because they somehow seem insignificant when set against a large fry-up, say, or a big slice of cake. Those liquid calories surely don't count in the same way, do they?

Perhaps this was true once upon a time, when all we really drank was tea, coffee, water, milk and perhaps some orange squash as a treat (i.e. the fifties!). But things are different now; all you have to do is go into your nearest express supermarket or petrol station, and there's a whole wall of fridges offering up everything from classic fizzy sodas to 'healthy' vitamin waters and sugar-stacked energy drinks.

When thinking about our overall nutrition, we simply cannot ignore what we consume in liquid form; for some of us, it will be a major source of sugar and calorie intake. A recent YouGov survey established that 62% of adults regularly purchase soft drinks.[56] Admittedly, this did include bottled water, but the consumption of shop-bought drinks is certainly a well-established habit in this country. Another survey by the fitness company PureGym found that the average Brit consumes 322 cans of sugary drinks a year, equivalent to 2 litres a week.[57] To put this in context, 2 litres of a well-known carbonated soft drink contains 840 calories and 215g of sugar, so it's certainly not insignificant.

Perhaps you aren't guzzling fizzy drinks, but let's look at coffee. If you regularly buy your flat white at a well-known coffee outlet, that's 119 calories a pop and 8g of sugar before you've even glanced at the muffins. Again, this is not insignificant when you look at our national consumption habits. A 2020 survey by the World Coffee Portal estimated that more than one fifth (21%) of consumers drink four or more cups of coffee per day.[58] Coffee is known to have some health benefits (see below), but in the context of calorie and sugar intake, it still counts.

And all this is before we've even considered booze. Statistics are stark. According to the latest government figures, in England 82% of adults drank alcohol in the past 12 months, with 49% of adults drinking at least once a week, and over 40% drinking more than the recommended 14 units a week.[59] If you are having difficulty imagining 14 units, that's about a bottle and a half of wine, which at an average 13% alcohol, contains over 1,000 calories.

The takeaway message is clear: we need to think about our drinks when it comes to our overall nutrition.

I'm confused about coffee! One minute it's good for you, the next minute it's not

Coffee contains caffeine, a stimulant, which is responsible for helping us feel awake and alert. In the past, caffeine has been linked to adverse health outcomes like heart disease and even cancer. But more recent studies have come out in favour of coffee consumption, including one by Queen Mary University of London, which found that having up to three cups of coffee a day has a protective effect on heart health.[60] It is also associated with a reduction in overall mortality rate and the risk of stroke.

As I've tried to establish throughout this book, we are all unique. We all have different responses to what we put in our bodies, so there's a certain amount of experimentation required. Your personal sweet spot for coffee might be just one cup. Certainly, I know people who, if they have more than this, can feel jittery and over-stimulated, while others can easily have four or five cups with no negative effects. As caffeine can stay in the system for up to seven hours, though, it's advisable to avoid it later in the day, or it can have a negative impact on your quality of sleep.

Other than the effects of caffeine, coffee can be a good inclusion in your diet because it contains polyphenols and a reasonable amount of fibre (around 0.5g per cup), and these are good for our hearts, brains and gut health. So if you enjoy your coffee, crack on – just be mindful of what else you put into it. Black coffee or coffee with a splash of milk is fine; once you get into elaborate milky coffees or those with syrups or toppings, any benefits from the coffee will most likely be outweighed by the additional calorie/sugar intake.

I've heard that some alcohol, especially red wine, is good for you

The original theory that red wine is good for heart health comes from the idea of the 'French Paradox', a term used to explain the relatively low incidence of cardiovascular disease in the French population despite a high-fat diet. This was thought to be attributable to the regular consumption of red wine, which contains heart-healthy polyphenols. More recent evidence on whether some alcohol consumption is beneficial for health is mixed. A number of studies have found some heart-health benefits associated with moderate alcohol intake,[61] whereas the most recent findings by researchers at Massachusetts General Hospital indicated that alcohol intake at all levels was linked with higher risks of cardiovascular disease.[62]

And then there are the social benefits of having a drink to consider. A recent observational study from researchers in Germany questioned over 600 people over the age of 60. They found that the drinkers among them were slimmer, happier and more mobile than their teetotal and low-drinking counterparts.[63] One explanation may be that higher alcohol consumption leads to elevated mood, enhanced sociability and reduced stress.

Drinks recap

- Don't ignore the nutritional impact of what you drink. It all counts and needs to be considered in the context of our overall diet.
- Soft drinks can contain large amounts of sugar and calories and are best avoided.
- Moderate coffee (and tea) intake is fine but have it black or with just a splash of milk, and no sugar.
- Consuming 14 units or less of alcohol a week is considered safe but you need to consider you own personal health risk factors.

As with the coffee question, there is no 'one-size-fits-all' set of rules when it comes to alcohol. The current UK guidelines advise having no more than 14 units of alcohol a week but we each have a unique set of risk factors that can potentially affect our long-term health outcomes. It's important to take this into account when considering your own alcohol consumption.

Ten easy ways to think about what you drink

1. **Reduce soft drinks in favour of plain water.** Carrying a water bottle with you throughout the day will reduce your reliance on shop-bought drinks. See also the tips for staying hydrated on page 57.

2. **Eat fruit, don't drink it.** Fruit juices may seem a healthier option, and indeed they can provide some vitamins and minerals, but the sugar content can be high, and so can the calorie content. Better to make your own healthy smoothies or eat the fruit whole, as nature intended.

3. **Ditch the lattes.** Ideally drink coffee black, or with just a splash of milk, and no sugar so the calorie count doesn't rack up.

4. **Start the day a different way.** You don't have to have coffee as a 'pick-me-up' in the morning; try making a healthy infusion, such as the Zingy 'Get Going' Morning Tea (page 246) instead.

5. **Skip the evening glass of wine.** Break your evening wine habit by switching to a new healthy one, like the Sleeping Potion on page 253, which contains sleep-promoting hormones and minerals, including tryptophan, melatonin and magnesium.

6. **Stick to the 'rule of three'.** Have alcohol on no more than three days a week, and have no more than three drinks when you do drink. Remember the recommended limit is 14 units of alcohol per week.

7. **Dilute your alcoholic drinks.** Opt for a more diluted alcoholic drink, such as a spritzer or shandy, or add lots of ice to a gin and tonic. Another good tactic is to alternate a glass of water with each alcoholic drink.

8. **Stick to NOLO in the week.** There are some excellent NOLO (no- and low-alcohol) products on the market now that tick the psychological 'I'm having a drink' box without the unwelcome after-effects.

9. **Make a mocktail.** Alcohol-free options don't have to be dull. When friends come over, try my Alcohol-free White Sangria (page 250) or Hydrating Watermelon Mocktail (page 251).

10. **Join the kombucha club.** Sparkling kombucha, which you can now buy in corked bottles like sparkling wine, is a great alcohol alternative with added gut-health benefits.

The Recipes

And now for the best bit: the food! We've covered a lot of nutritional theory and healthy-eating recommendations, but in the end, supercharging your diet comes down to what you do in the kitchen. To make this easier, I've created recipes for each of the 'ten easy ways' categories, grouped as follows:

1. Complex carbohydrates

2. Lean protein

3. Healthy fats

4. Fibre-rich

5. Gut health

6. Five-a-day

7. Vitamins and minerals

8. Lower-calorie meals

9. Smart snacks and sweet stuff

10. Healthy drinks

Even though a recipe has been assigned to one category, that's not to say it isn't applicable in many of the others – one that's very fibre-rich is no doubt also good for the gut, and a recipe that's in the five-a-day section will certainly contain lots of vitamins and minerals. Suffice to say, if you are cooking a range of recipes across all the categories, you can be sure you are getting a good balance of healthy macros and a wide range of all the micronutrients you need.

Interpreting the nutritional information

Under the recipe title, you will see the following designators if they are applicable:

VG (vegan)

VE (lacto-ovo vegetarian)

DF (dairy-free)

GF (gluten-free)

The nutritional information provided for each recipe is calculated based on the stated serving size; so if a recipe serves two, then the nutritional information per serving is based on half the quantity produced by the recipe.

Here's an example of the nutritional information for a recipe and how to interpret the information:

Nutrients (per serving)

Calories 369   *Protein* 13.9g (14%)

Total fat / saturated fat / omega-3 13.1g (30%) / 4.0g / 0.1g

Total carbs / sugar / fibre 54.7g (56%) / 29.8g / 6.2g

Vitamins and minerals B2, B6, B12, potassium

- The total calorie count per serving for this recipe is 369.

- A serving contains 13.9g of protein, which is 14% of the total calorie content of that serving. The RNI for protein is 45g per day for a woman and 56g per day for a man.

- A serving contains 13.1g of total fat, which is 30% of the total calorie content of that serving. Of this, 4.0g is saturated fat and 0.1g is omega-3 fatty acids. The RNI for saturated fat is 20g per day for a woman and 30g per day for a man. There

A word on salt

I don't specifically give information on the salt content of the recipes, because when cooking from scratch, the use of some salt for seasoning is no reason for concern from a health perspective. If you have been advised to reduce the salt in your diet by your doctor, then any added salt can be completely omitted if you wish; this will obviously affect the flavour of the dish, so you may wish to increase other flavouring elements, like lemon juice, herbs and spices.

is no official RNI for omega-3, but a good target is around 1.5g per day.

- A serving contains 54.7g of total carbohydrates, which is 56% of the total calorie content of that serving. Of this, 29.8g is sugar and 6.2g is fibre. The RNI for 'free sugar' is 30g per day, so while this sugar count may seem high, these are intrinsic sugars, as I use very small amounts of free sugars in my recipes. The RNI for fibre is 30g per day.

- The vitamins and minerals listed are just the headline micronutrients for the recipe. There will most certainly be others, as the recipes are designed for maximum nutrition, but there isn't the space to give a complete nutritional breakdown of every single micronutrient for each recipe. For more detailed information on the best food sources of each micronutrient, refer back to pages 84–5.

My hero ingredients

Most of the ingredients I use in these recipes are everyday ones that you will be familiar with. There are certain ingredients that crop up very regularly because they enhance not only the nutritional value but also the flavour of the recipes. I call these my 'hero' ingredients.

Greek yogurt – I use the 5% Fage brand Greek yogurt. You can use any make you like, but be sure to use live yogurt; some of the 'Greek-style' yogurts don't deliver the same gut-health benefits.

Date syrup – I do use honey and maple syrup from time to time, but my absolute favourite sweetener is date syrup. I use the Biona brand, which is made from whole, organic dates, because it has a lovely, rich flavour.

Mixed seeds – You can buy packets of mixed seeds in all supermarkets now. Choosing mixed seeds increases your plant-food count, which is good for gut health, rather than sticking to a single variety. I use them in many recipes, but they are also great just toasted in a pan and sprinkled over whatever sweet and savoury dishes you fancy.

Pre-cooked pouches of lentils and grains – I keep a wide variety of these in my cupboard, and they're an absolute saviour on a busy weeknight. Most supermarkets do their own versions now, but I usually buy the Merchant Gourmet brand. For best results, I tip them into a sieve and pour over a kettle of boiling water to refresh them. Use a fork to break up any clumps and then run cold water over them if they are needed cold or at room temperature for a salad.

Tins of beans and chickpeas – If you have the time or forethought to pre-soak and cook beans and chickpeas, then by all means do so; it will work out cheaper that way. I, however, am not that person, and so I regularly resort to the tinned versions, which you will see cropping up often in the recipes that follow.

Organic stock cubes – I have all the different types of Kallo organic stock cubes, but my most oft-used are the vegetable ones. They're an absolute boon and add extra depth of flavour to many, many of the dishes in this book. Stock up!

The Recipes

Apple cider vinegar – Apple cider vinegar, or ACV as it is also known, is my go-to vinegar, not just for its versatility, but because if you buy one with live cultures, sometimes referred to as 'the mother', then you are getting a very useful hit of probiotics for good gut health.

Spices – My most-used spices are ground cumin, ground coriander, ground turmeric, chilli powder, dried red chilli flakes and ground cinnamon. You will find others used in this book, but these are the ones you can't do without.

Fresh herbs – Think about adding fresh herbs to dishes wherever you can. The ones I use most are coriander, mint and flat-leaf parsley. They are an excellent way to increase the number of plant foods on your plate and it's easy to grow your own in pots.

Lemons – The number of lemons I get through in a week is astonishing. In my view, there is very little that doesn't benefit from a squeeze of lemon juice. In fact, I call it the third seasoning, as a bowl of lemons sits on my countertop next to the salt and pepper grinders. If you make something and it tastes a bit flat, some acidity from lemon juice is often all that it needs.

Extra virgin olive oil – For cold use in dressings and for drizzling, you can't get better than a really good-quality extra virgin olive oil. For cooking, you can use the more refined 'light' olive oil, which has a neutral flavour.

Organic rapeseed oil – When a high-smoke-point oil is required for cooking, I favour a good-quality, organic rapeseed oil. It is high in unsaturated fat, contains vitamins E and K, and has a good omega-3 to omega-6 ratio, which is beneficial for heart health.

Sea salt flakes and fine sea salt – Have both types of salt available when cooking; fine sea salt is better when a specific measurement is given, but if the instruction is simply 'a good pinch', I like to use flakes. Flakes are also good for finishing a dish when seasoning is required at the end.

Black pepper – Essential and used throughout. Make sure you always use freshly ground; the pre-ground stuff just doesn't have the same punch.

Additional notes on the recipes

1. A weight reference is given for some ingredients for guidance where it is important for the balance of the recipe, or where the size of an ingredient can vary greatly, e.g. '1 small sweet potato (300g)'. If the weight isn't specified, e.g. '1 small red onion' then you can use your judgement: it won't negatively impact the final result if you are a bit over or under.

2. The preparation required for the ingredient is stated next to that ingredient, so it will say, '2 garlic cloves, finely grated'. I advise getting out all the ingredients and doing any required preparation before you start on the main method.

3. Where a recipe requires 'neutral' oil, this can be any high-smoke-point oil that has a neutral flavour. I favour organic rapeseed oil, as explained above, but you could use light olive oil. I don't recommend soy bean, sunflower or corn oils, as they are very high in omega-6.

4. All oven temperatures given assume you have a fan-assisted oven. Increase the temperature by 20°C if you don't.

Recipe Listing

Complex carbohydrates

Lean protein

The Recipes

The Recipes

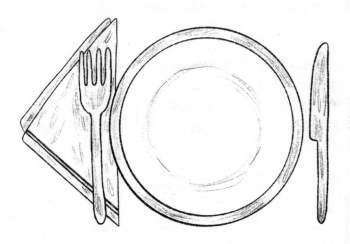

COMPLEX CARBOHYDRATES

Wholegrain Granola

VE, DF, GF (use GF-certified oats)

I put a new granola recipe in each of my books because I'm obsessed with the stuff. I'm particularly happy with this one because it's so simple, and there are no added sugars, nor any additional oil. The sweetness and crunch comes from whole dates whizzed up with egg whites; this mixture coats the oats, seeds and nuts, and then they're all baked to a golden crisp. Enjoy!

Prep: 10 mins   Cooking: 30 mins   Servings: 10 × 50g

200g rolled oats
100g mixed seeds (sunflower, pumpkin, flax, sesame)
50g flaked almonds
1 teaspoon ground cinnamon (optional)
4 pitted Medjool dates*
2 egg whites

Preheat the oven to 150°C/gas mark 3½. Line a large baking tray with parchment.

Put the oats, seeds and almonds in a large bowl. Add the cinnamon if using, and mix well.

In a high-speed blender, whizz up the dates and egg whites until they are fully combined and a bit frothy. Pour this mixture into the bowl

* If you can't find plump Medjool dates, you can use other varieties, but they may need to be soaked in water for an hour or two first in order to blend well with the egg whites.

with the dry ingredients, using a spatula to make sure you scrape it all out. Use a metal fork to thoroughly mix the date mixture into the dry ingredients until they are fully coated and a little damp.

Spread the mixture on the tray and bake for 20 minutes. Remove from the oven and use a spatula to gently release the granola from the parchment, breaking it up into chunks. Return to the oven for a further 10 minutes, then turn off the oven and allow the granola to cool completely in the oven to make sure it's really dry and crunchy.

Store in an airtight container. Will keep for 3 to 4 weeks.

Nutrients (per serving)
Calories 195   *Protein* 7.6g (14%)
Total fat / saturated fat / omega-3 9.0g (38%) / 1.0g / 0.4g
Total carbs / sugar / fibre 23.5g (48%) / 6.8g / 4.5g
Vitamins and minerals B1, E, magnesium

Wake-up Smoothie

VE, GF (use GF-certified oats)

This smoothie is all about getting going in the morning: complex carbs for slow-release energy, healthy fats for satiety and that all-important caffeine fix provided by a teaspoon of instant coffee added to the mix. This recipe uses frozen bananas, so when you have a couple of overripe ones, peel, chop and freeze, and they are ready to go.

Prep: 5 mins   Cooking: 0 mins   Serves: 1

- 1 large banana, chopped and frozen
- 1 tablespoon peanut butter (or other nut butter)
- 1 tablespoon rolled oats
- 200ml semi-skimmed milk (can also use a non-dairy milk)
- 1 teaspoon instant coffee

Place all the ingredients in a high-speed blender and whizz together for 60 seconds until smooth. Add a drop more milk if it's not moving or if you like it a bit runnier. Enjoy straight away.

Nutrients (per serving)

Calories 369   *Protein* 13.9g (14%)

Total fat / saturated fat / omega-3 13.1g (30%) / 4.0g / 0.1g

Total carbs / sugar / fibre 54.7g (56%) / 29.8g / 6.2g

Vitamins and minerals B2, B6, B12, potassium

Vanilla and Cardamom Porridge

VE, GF (use GF-certified oats)

This spiced porridge packs in your complex carbs early in the day so your body can make the most of the slow-release energy they provide.

Prep: 5 mins   Cooking: 10 mins   Serves: 2

100g rolled oats
400ml semi-skimmed milk
2 tablespoons raisins
½ teaspoon ground cinnamon
½ teaspoon vanilla extract
1 tablespoon date syrup
3 cardamom pods, gently crushed
pinch of salt

Place all the ingredients in a medium saucepan over a medium heat. Bring to the boil, then reduce the heat to low and simmer for ten minutes, stirring occasionally. Eat while piping hot.

Nutrients (per serving)

Calories 366   *Protein* 15.6g (16%)

Total fat / saturated fat / omega-3 7.5g (18%) / 3.1g / 0.0g

Total carbs / sugar / fibre 60.1g (66%) / 23.6g / 6.3g

Vitamins and minerals B12, magnesium, zinc

Spicy Sweet Potato Soup

VG, VE, DF, GF

Put aside any carb prejudice you may have; this soup is carb-packed and low-cal – yes, it's possible! This recipe makes five servings, so if you make it at the weekend, you've got lunch sorted for the week. All those complex carbs will give you energy as well as delivering a bonanza of micronutrients.

Prep: 15 mins   Cooking: 25 mins   Serves: 5

1 tablespoon light olive oil
1 small onion, diced
2 garlic cloves, finely grated
1 tablespoon finely grated fresh root ginger
1 teaspoon ground cumin
1 teaspoon ground coriander
1 teaspoon ground turmeric
1 small sweet potato (300g), peeled and finely diced
1 small cauliflower head (300g), chopped into tiny florets
400g tin chopped tomatoes
1 litre (1¾ pints) vegetable stock, made from 2 cubes
salt and freshly ground black pepper
400g tin black lentils, rinsed and drained
150g cavolo nero or other leafy green, roughly chopped

Heat the oil in a large saucepan over a medium heat. Add the onions and gently fry to soften. After about 5 minutes, add the garlic, ginger and spices, and fry for a further minute or two. Add the sweet potato and cauliflower and stir well into the spicy mixture, then add the tomatoes and stock and season well with salt and pepper. Bring to the boil, then reduce the heat to low and simmer for 20 minutes.

Add the lentils and cavolo nero, and simmer for a few more minutes. The soup is now ready to serve. If you prefer a smoother texture, you can give it a blitz with a hand-blender.

Nutrients (per serving)
Calories 187 *Protein* 7.6g (12%)
Total fat / saturated fat / omega-3 4.0g (19%) / 0.5g / 0.3g
Total carbs / sugar / fibre 33.5g (69%) / 9.2g / 9.0g
Vitamins and minerals A, C, K, copper, magnesium

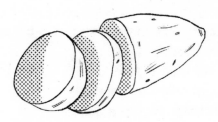

Roasted Roots with Feta and Mint

VE, GF

I've done various versions of this recipe over the years, but I think this pared-down one is my absolute favourite. It's bold enough to stand alone as a glorious lunch, but it also makes a super-tasty side dish for any grilled meat or fish. I'd recommend roasting the veg earlier in the day so they can come down to room temperature for when you want to serve.

Prep: 10 mins   Cooking: 40 mins   Serves: 4

500g sweet potatoes, peeled and chopped into chunks
250g raw beetroot, peeled and roughly chopped
250g carrots, peeled and roughly chopped
2 large red onions (300g), roughly chopped
1 tablespoon extra virgin olive oil
salt and freshly ground black pepper
20g pine nuts
1 tablespoon pomegranate molasses (or ½ tablespoon honey)
1 tablespoon red wine vinegar
a small handful of picked mint leaves
100g feta, crumbled

Preheat the oven to 200°C/gas mark 7.

Place the sweet potatoes, beetroot, carrots and onions in a roasting tin and drizzle over the olive oil. Toss well to coat and season with salt and pepper. Roast for 40 minutes, giving it all a good stir halfway through. Remove from the oven and leave to cool to room temperature.

Meanwhile, toast the pine nuts in a hot, non-stick frying pan for a couple of minutes until golden.

Place the cooled roasted vegetables in a nice bowl. In a small jug or bowl, mix together the pomegranate molasses and red wine vinegar, then pour this over the roasted vegetables and toss well to coat. Sprinkle over the mint leaves, crumbled feta and toasted pine nuts, and serve.

Nutrients (per serving)

Calories 279   *Protein* 8.3g (10%)

Total fat / saturated fat / omega-3 12.7g (40%) / 4.6g / 0.1g

Total carbs / sugar / fibre 36.1g (50%) / 21.8g / 8.6g

Vitamins and minerals A, B2, B6, calcium, magnesium, zinc

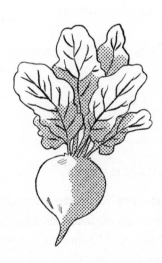

Quick Spicy Bulgur Salad
VG, VE, DF

I absolutely love the flavours of the Middle East and bulgur wheat is a brilliant wholegrain ingredient that offers a healthier alternative to couscous. It's put to great use in this riff on tabbouleh, made with lots of parsley, but it's the spicy dressing that takes it to the next level. A fab salad for a barbecue, this also works well as a side dish any day of the week.

Prep: 10 mins   Cooking: 10 mins   Serves: 4

120g bulgur wheat
salt and freshly ground black pepper
60g flat-leaf parsley, tough stalks removed, finely chopped
1 medium red onion (100g), diced
1 medium ripe tomato (100g), diced
30g raisins

For the dressing
1 tablespoon extra virgin olive oil
1 tablespoon harissa paste
1 tablespoon date syrup (or maple syrup)
juice of ½ lemon
1 teaspoon ground cumin
1 teaspoon ground turmeric

Cook the bulgur wheat according to the packet instructions, then fluff with a fork and allow to cool completely.

Make the dressing by mixing together all the dressing ingredients in a bowl. Pour this over the cooled bulgur wheat. Using a spatula, mix well until all the bulgur is well coated. Season with plenty of salt and pepper.

The Recipes

Add the flat-leaf parsley, onion, tomato and raisins and stir to combine, then serve.

> **Nutrients (per serving)**
> *Calories* 202   *Protein* 5.5g (10%)
> *Total fat / saturated fat / omega-3* 4.3g (18%) / 0.6g / 0.0g
> *Total carbs / sugar / fibre* 39.5g (72%) / 10.8g / 5.8g
> *Vitamins and minerals* A, C, K, magnesium, manganese, phosphorus

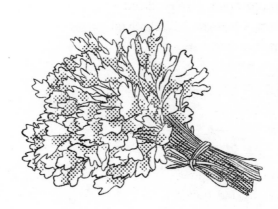

Squash, Spinach and Potato Curry

VG, VE, DF, GF

There's a bit of prep to do here to get all the veggies ready, but it only takes about 30 minutes to cook, so as curries go, it's pretty speedy. The focus here is on energy-giving complex carbs, so make a big batch, have some for dinner and enjoy the leftovers for a sustaining lunch the next day. It's rather nice with a blob of thick Greek yogurt on top, but I'll leave this as an option.

Prep: 15 mins   Cooking: 35 mins   Serves: 4

1 tablespoon neutral oil
1 teaspoon mustard seeds
1 small onion, diced
2 garlic cloves, finely grated
1 tablespoon finely grated fresh root ginger
1 teaspoon hot chilli powder
2 teaspoons ground cumin
2 teaspoons ground coriander
1 teaspoon ground turmeric
500ml vegetable stock, made from 1 cube
500g potatoes, peeled and chopped into 2–3cm cubes
500g butternut squash, peeled, deseeded and cut into
    2–3cm cubes
400ml can light coconut milk
150g baby spinach leaves, rinsed
juice of 1 lime
20g salted peanuts, chopped
a small handful of coriander leaves, chopped

Heat the oil in a large saucepan or wok over a medium heat. Add the mustard seeds. When they start to pop, add the onion and fry gently for a few minutes to soften, then add the garlic and ginger and cook for a further minute. Add the chilli powder, cumin, ground coriander and turmeric. Mix everything together well, and let it cook for another minute, adding a splash of the stock if it's sticking.

Add the potatoes and butternut squash and stir, then add the coconut milk and the stock. Bring to the boil, then reduce the heat to low and simmer for 30 minutes until the potatoes and butternut squash are tender.

Add the spinach and lime juice and gently stir until the spinach has wilted down. Serve with a sprinkle of chopped peanuts and coriander leaves on top.

Nutrients (per serving)
Calories 292   *Protein* 7.0g (7%)
Total fat / saturated fat / omega-3 14.4g (42%) / 7.8g / 0.4g
Total carbs / sugar / fibre 39.1g (51%) / 6.7g / 5.1g
Vitamins and minerals A, B6, C, magnesium, manganese, iron

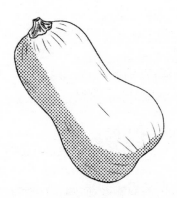

Giant Couscous Risotto with Chicken and Chorizo

DF

If you are a risotto fan, you'll love the texture of this oven-baked version, which requires no stirring. In the interests of health and calories, while this is cooked with the skin on the chicken to retain moisture, I recommend removing it when eating it, because it really just adds a load of extra saturated animal fat to the dish that you can do without. Needless to say, there's plenty of protein on the plate here, and the couscous is a good source of fibre. If you have trouble sourcing wholemeal couscous, you can use brown rice instead, but the cooking time will be longer.

Prep: 15 mins   Cooking: 45 mins   Serves: 4

  8 skin-on boneless chicken thighs (1kg)
  1 large red onion, sliced
  80g chorizo, peeled and chopped into semi-circles
  2 red peppers, deseeded and sliced
  2 garlic cloves, finely grated
  1 teaspoon paprika
  ½ teaspoon hot chilli powder
  1 tablespoon tomato purée
  400ml chicken stock from a cube
  salt and freshly ground black pepper
  150g dried giant wholemeal couscous (or brown rice)

Preheat the oven to 200°C/gas mark 7.

Heat a large frying pan over a medium heat, then add the chicken pieces and cook for a few minutes on each side until a little browned. You'll probably have to do this in two batches. Remove the chicken to a plate lined with kitchen paper and discard any fat in the pan.

Add the onion and chorizo to the pan and fry for 3–4 minutes until the chorizo has released its oil and the onion has softened. Then add the peppers and garlic and continue to fry for a few more minutes until the peppers are starting to soften. Add the paprika and chilli powder and mix well.

Add the tomato purée to the stock and mix well to dissolve, then pour this mixture into the pan. Season well with salt and pepper.

Take a large glass baking dish and pour in the couscous, spreading it evenly over the base. Add the contents of the frying pan to the dish, distributing it over the couscous, then arrange the chicken pieces, skin-side up, on top. Bake for 30 minutes.

Remove from the oven, set the chicken pieces aside on a plate and stir the couscous mixture beneath; it should be like a risotto. If it's too liquid, return to the oven for a further 5–10 minutes (cover the chicken to keep it warm in the meantime).

To serve, remove the skin from the chicken pieces and place on top of the creamy giant couscous risotto. Alternatively, you can shred the chicken and stir it through.

Nutrients (per serving)

Calories 561   *Protein* 59.7g (45%)

Total fat / saturated fat / omega-3 18.7g (30%) / 5.7g / 0.2g

Total carbs / sugar / fibre 35.0g (25%) / 4.8g / 4.0g

Vitamins and minerals A, B3, B6, C, phosphorus, selenium, zinc

---

LEAN PROTEIN

Protein Power Smoothie

VE, GF

Time was when cottage cheese was the dieter's food of choice, but did you know it's actually an excellent source of lean protein? Here, it's put to good use in a smoothie. Surprisingly, cherries also contain some protein, but if you don't have any, you can use any frozen berries. This smoothie also delivers a good hit of plant-based omega-3 in the form of ALA. Quick tip: store any extra avocado in a bowl of water in the fridge for up to a day. This will stop it going brown.

Prep: 5 mins   Cooking: 0 mins   Serves: 1 (generously)

150g cottage cheese
100g frozen cherries (or
   other berries)
½ ripe banana, peeled
¼ ripe avocado, peeled
2 teaspoons honey

1 tablespoon ground flaxseeds
   (use pre-ground flaxseeds
   or grind them in a coffee
   grinder)
200ml semi-skimmed milk

Place all the ingredients in a blender and whizz until completely smooth. Enjoy straight away.

Nutrients (per serving)

Calories 422   *Protein* 28.7g (28%)

Total fat / saturated fat / omega-3 13.2g (27%) / 4.5g / 1.7g

Total carbs / sugar / fibre 51.5g (45%) / 39.3g / 7.3g

Vitamins and minerals B2, B6, B12, calcium, magnesium,
   selenium

Prawn and Pak Choy Omelette

DF, GF

If you are thinking prawns and eggs are a bit of an odd combo, this is like a Chinese-style prawn egg-fried rice without the rice! There's absolutely oodles of protein here, so it's an ideal start to the day, and you can balance it up with a slice of your favourite bread.

Prep: 5 mins   Cooking: 5 mins   Serves: 1

2 eggs
½ teaspoon neutral oil
½ teaspoon sesame oil
100g raw tiger prawns
handful of pak choy leaves
     (50g), chopped

2 spring onions, finely sliced
salt and freshly ground black
     pepper

Whisk together the eggs in a small bowl. Heat the oils in a medium-sized non-stick frying pan over a medium heat. Add the prawns and cook for approximately 30 seconds on each side until pink. Add the pak choy and spring onions and cook for a further minute until wilted. Pour over the eggs and sprinkle some salt and pepper over the top. Cook for a couple of minutes until golden, then flip to cook on the other side for 1 minute. If you prefer a runnier omelette, just cook on one side and then, when the eggs are nearly cooked on the upper side, fold in half. Serve straight away.

Nutrients (per serving)

Calories 285   *Protein* 11.9g (48%)

Total fat / saturated fat / omega-3 5.2g (46%) / 2.7g / 0.4g

Total carbs / sugar / fibre 1.4g (6%) / 1.7g / 1.3g

Vitamins and minerals A, B2, B12, K, calcium, iodine,
     magnesium, selenium

Coriander Chicken Soup

DF, GF

This soup is absolutely gorgeous, so if you are in need of some filling, sustaining protein, this is the healthy way to go. It's actually a twist on a recipe called Aguadito, a Peruvian dish, which was very popular in my first book, but I've pumped in even more protein in the form of kidney beans, which gives it a distinctly Mexican vibe.

Prep: 10 mins   Cooking: 25 mins   Serves: 2

1 small onion, roughly chopped
1 garlic clove, roughly chopped
1 large green chilli, deseeded and roughly chopped
30g fresh coriander, leaves and stalks, roughly chopped
juice of 1 lime
1 tablespoon extra virgin olive oil
40g quinoa, rinsed
500ml chicken stock from a cube
150g pre-cooked chicken breast, shredded
130g tinned red kidney beans (drained weight)
salt and freshly ground black pepper

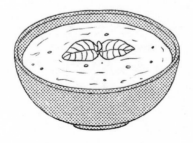

Place the onion, garlic, chilli, coriander and lime juice in a food processor and blitz to a salsa-like consistency.

Heat the oil in a large saucepan over a medium heat. Add the contents of the food processor and gently sauté for about 2 minutes. Add the quinoa and stock, then reduce the heat and simmer for 15 minutes.

Now add the chicken and beans. Mix well, taste, and season with salt and pepper. Simmer for a further 5 minutes or so, then serve. If at any point there's not enough liquid, just top up with a little extra water.

Nutrients (per serving)

Calories 311   *Protein* 30.2g (39%)

Total fat / saturated fat / omega-3 10.6g (30%) / 1.9g / 0.1g

Total carbs / sugar / fibre 24.6g (31%) / 6.4g / 5.3g

Vitamins and minerals B3, B6, C, copper, phosphorus, selenium

---

Mushroom and Lentil Masala

VE, GF

I know you will look at this recipe and your immediate reaction will be 'too many ingredients', but please don't be put off! Most of the list are simply spices you'll already have in your cupboard, and you just need to bung them in the blender to make a paste. The curry itself is so simple, and it's got those lovely rich masala flavours, along with a big whack of plant-based protein and fibre. Serve with brown basmati rice or wholegrain pitas.

Prep: 15 mins   Cooking: 35 mins   Serves: 4

1 tablespoon neutral oil
250g onions, finely sliced
450g mushrooms, chopped into chunks
250g red peppers, chopped into chunks
400g tin lentils, drained and rinsed
400g tin chopped tomatoes
2 tablespoons tomato purée
100g plain yogurt
small handful of coriander leaves, to serve

For the paste
5 garlic cloves, roughly chopped
15g fresh root ginger, peeled and roughly chopped
2 large red chillies, deseeded and roughly chopped
2 teaspoons ground cumin
2 teaspoons ground coriander
1 teaspoon ground turmeric
1 teaspoon garam masala
4 cardamom pods, seeds only
½ teaspoon salt

The Recipes

Place all the curry paste ingredients in a blender along with 5 tablespoons water and whizz on low for 20 seconds, then scrape down the sides of the blender and blend on high for a further 20–30 seconds until it's nice and smooth.

Heat the oil in a large saucepan or flat-based wok over a low–medium heat. Add the onions and gently sauté for 10 minutes, stirring from time to time, until nice and soft. Remove the onions from the pan and set aside on a plate. Add the mushrooms and peppers to the pan, increase the heat to medium and sauté for 5 minutes or so, until the mushrooms are starting to colour. Remove the mushrooms and peppers from the pan and set aside on the plate with the onions.

Now add the spice paste to the pan and fry for 1 minute before returning all the vegetables to the pan and stirring well to combine. Add the lentils, tomatoes and tomato purée, then top up with 500ml water. Increase the heat and bring to the boil, then reduce the heat to low and simmer for 15 minutes.

Just before serving, stir through the plain yogurt and reheat gently, but don't boil. Serve with a scattering of chopped coriander leaves over the top.

Nutrients (per serving)

Calories 216   *Protein* 14.0g (21%)

Total fat / saturated fat / omega-3 5.0g (20%) / 0.8g / 0.3g

Total carbs / sugar / fibre 33.7g (59%) / 9.5g / 10.4g

Vitamins and minerals B1, B2, C, iron, potassium, zinc

Wild Salmon Poke Bowl

DF

You might not feel too confident handling raw fish – indeed, I tend to think it's best left to the sushi masters – but really what we are dealing with here is more of an Asian-style ceviche. The beauty of this dish is you can vary it according to what you have available veggies-wise; the only thing you absolutely must have is a really good-quality piece of fresh, wild salmon – and remember to look for that all-important blue MSC mark for sustainability. As you'd suspect, a bowl of this has bags of protein and ticks your omega-3 box.

Prep: 15 mins   Cooking: 3 mins   Serves: 2

250g pouch of pre-cooked wholegrain rice
1 teaspoon sesame oil
salt
2 tablespoons soy sauce (use tamari to make it GF)
juice of ½ lime
1 teaspoon finely grated fresh root ginger
2 spring onions, finely sliced
200g fillet wild salmon, skin removed, sliced into
    1–2cm cubes
4 tablespoons rice vinegar (or other light-coloured vinegar)
2 teaspoons honey
100g cucumber, halved then cut into semi-circles
75g edamame beans*
1 teaspoon sesame seeds
1 medium carrot (150g), peeled and sliced into thin strips
    (julienne), or grated
½ avocado, peeled, stoned and sliced

* You can buy frozen, podded edamame beans in the supermarket. Just
defrost in boiling water before use.

The Recipes

Boil a kettle of water and empty the pouch of rice into a sieve. Holding it over the sink, pour over the boiling water, then run the cold tap over the rice and drain thoroughly.

Place the refreshed rice in a bowl and pour over the sesame oil. Add a pinch of salt and mix well.

In a separate bowl, mix together the soy sauce, lime juice, ginger and spring onions. Add the salmon cubes and stir to ensure the fish is completely soaked in the dressing. Set aside.

In a third bowl, whisk together the rice vinegar and honey. Add the cucumber slices and toss to coat, then leave to marinate.

Finally, toast the sesame seeds in a hot, dry frying pan for a few minutes until golden.

Now it's time to assemble the dish. Take two serving bowls and divide the rice equally between them. Top with the salmon and arrange the cucumber, edamame beans, carrot and avocado around the sides. If there's any of the fish marinade left in the bowl, drizzle it over the top, then finish with the toasted sesame seeds and serve.

Nutrients (per serving)
Calories 501   *Protein* 32.4g (26%)
Total fat / saturated fat / omega-3 19.6g (34%) / 3.2g / 1.5g
Total carbs / sugar / fibre 40.2g (40%) / 10.3g / 9.6g
Vitamins and minerals A, B vitamins, D, magnesium,
    manganese, selenium

Baked Chicken with Dijon Mustard and Mushrooms

GF

Credit where credit's due: this dish is adapted from a recipe by one of my favourite food writers, Diana Henry, in her awesome book *From the Oven to the Table*. I've made a few health tweaks, of course, namely adding mushrooms (which, incidentally, are a good source of plant protein and also do a great job of absorbing the delicious sauce). I've also swapped out the original vermouth for apple cider vinegar. I hope Diana won't mind! Serve with a dressed green salad and brown basmati rice. To reduce calories and saturated fat, remove the chicken skin before eating.

Prep: 10 mins   Cooking: 40 mins   Serves: 4

    250g chestnut mushrooms, quartered
    4 tablespoons Dijon mustard
    1 tablespoon extra virgin olive oil
    2 tablespoons apple cider vinegar
    2 garlic cloves, finely grated
    6 tablespoons light crème fraîche
    8 bone-in chicken thighs (with skin, but trim off any excess)
    salt and freshly ground black pepper

Preheat the oven to 190°C/gas mark 6½.

Place the mushrooms in a large glass baking dish (just large enough to comfortably fit the 8 chicken thighs).

In a bowl, combine the mustard, oil, vinegar and garlic with 4 tablespoons of the crème fraîche and 150ml water. Mix together until well combined – a mini whisk is great for this job. Add this mixture to the baking dish and mix well to coat the mushrooms.

The Recipes

Place the chicken thighs, skin-side up, into the dish, nestling them among the mushrooms so they sit in the nice creamy sauce. Season well with salt and pepper, making sure to get plenty on the chicken skin. Bake for 40 minutes.

Remove from the oven. Take out the chicken pieces and divide between four plates. Add the last 2 tablespoons of the crème fraîche to the mushroomy sauce in the baking dish and give it a good mix before spooning over the chicken and serving.

Nutrients (per serving)

Calories 751/451 with/without skin   *Protein* 52.9g (30%)

Total fat / saturated fat / omega-3 55.9g (66%) / 15.3g / 0.6g

Total carbs / sugar / fibre 7.3g (4%) / 0.9g / 2.1g

Vitamins and minerals B3, B6, B12, phosphorus, selenium, zinc

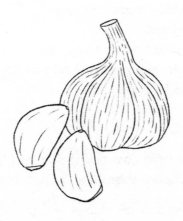

Sweet and Sour Pork Tenderloin with Braised Cabbage

DF

Pork tenderloin, or fillet, is my favourite weekday cut of pork, because it roasts so quickly in the oven and is really juicy and lean – it should be cooked through but still a little pink, unlike other cuts of pork. I've gone for a Chinese influence here, with a sweet and sour marinade and sesame oil to flavour the cabbage that sits underneath. Serve with some brown rice for a lovely balanced meal that delivers a load of lean protein.

Prep: 10 mins   Cooking: 30 mins   Serves: 4

1 small head white cabbage (600g)
3 tablespoons soy sauce (use tamari to make it GF)
1 tablespoon apple cider vinegar
1 tablespoon honey
1 tablespoon tomato purée
1 tablespoon finely grated fresh root ginger
2 garlic cloves, finely grated
½ teaspoon dried red chilli flakes (optional)
salt and freshly ground black pepper
2 teaspoons sesame oil
1 × 600g pork tenderloin or fillet

Preheat the oven to 200°C/gas mark 7 and boil a kettle of water.

Prepare the cabbage by removing any discoloured outer leaves, then cut it into large wedges and slice using the coarse slicer on your food processor. Place the sliced cabbage in a large bowl and pour over the boiling water. Leave to blanch while you make the marinade for the pork.

In a small bowl, mix together the soy sauce, apple cider vinegar, honey, tomato purée, ginger, garlic and chilli flakes, if using.

Drain the cabbage and place in a large glass baking dish. Season well with salt and pepper and drizzle over the sesame oil. Give it a good toss to coat and spread evenly over the base of the dish.

Place the pork fillet in the same bowl you used for the cabbage. Tip over the marinade, making sure the meat is completely coated. Place the fillet on top of the cabbage and pour any excess marinade back over the meat, then cover the baking dish with foil. You can cook this straight away and it will still taste great, or you can pop it in the fridge to marinade for an hour or two if you have time.

When you're ready to cook, place the foil-covered dish in the oven and roast for 30 minutes (5 minutes more if it's straight from the fridge). Remove from the oven and allow to rest for 10 minutes, then uncover. Remove the pork fillet and slice into finger-width slices. Give the cabbage a good mix to stir through all the juices. Divide the cabbage between four plates and top with the pork slices to serve.

Nutrients (per serving)
Calories 316 *Protein* 45.6g (60%)
Total fat / saturated fat / omega-3 6.9g (20%) / 1.8g / 0.1g
Total carbs / sugar / fibre 17.7g (20%) / 11.0g / 5.2g
Vitamins and minerals All the B vitamins, C, K, iron, selenium, zinc

Spicy Lamb Meatballs

DF, GF

Unless you are following a vegan or vegetarian diet, then eating good-quality meat occasionally delivers useful protein and micronutrients. If you can afford organic or high-welfare meat, it will ensure maximum benefit for both your health and the planet. These spicy, tomatoey meatballs are so yummy; serve with some wholegrain rice or wholemeal pasta and greens for a fabulous family-friendly mid-week meal.

Prep: 10 mins   Cooking: 20–25 mins   Serves: 4 x 5 meatballs

500g lean lamb mince
salt and freshly ground black pepper
1 tablespoon neutral oil
1 tablespoon white wine vinegar
400g tin chopped tomatoes
squeeze of lemon juice
½ teaspoon ground cinnamon
½ teaspoon dried red chilli flakes
1 teaspoon dried mixed herbs
1 tablespoon honey

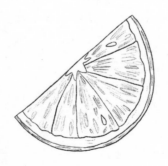

Place the lamb mince in a bowl, season well with salt and pepper and mix well. Divide into 20 × 25g portions and roll each one into a ball.

Heat the oil in a large, deep frying pan over a medium heat. Add the meatballs and brown on all sides for about 10 minutes, then remove from the pan and set aside on a plate to rest.

Discard any residual oil from the pan and return it to the heat. Add the vinegar, tomatoes, lemon juice, cinnamon, chilli flakes, dried herbs and honey, and season well with salt and pepper. Simmer for 5 minutes, then return the meatballs to the pan, along with any juices on the plate. Simmer all together for a further 5–10 minutes until the sauce is reduced to a nice thickness, then serve.

Nutrients (per serving)

Calories 280   *Protein* 26.0g (39%)

Total fat / saturated fat / omega-3 15.6g (49%) / 4.4g / 0.3g

Total carbs / sugar / fibre 9.3g (12%) / 7.2g / 2.4g

Vitamins and minerals B Vitamins, C, phosphorus, selenium, zinc

---

HEALTHY FATS

Omega-3 Smoothie

VG, VE, DF, GF

Here, I've put together the best plant-based omega-3 foods and paired them with sweet and delicious mango to make sure you are getting all those good fats. There's a massive 10g fibre per serving, too. The recipe doesn't include any sweetener as I think it is sweet enough, but you can add a little maple syrup or honey if you like.

Prep: 5 mins   Cooking: 0 mins   Serves: 1

4 walnut halves
10g chia seeds
10g flaxseeds

1 small banana, broken into a few pieces
100g frozen mango
200ml unsweetened soy milk

Place the walnuts, chia seeds and flaxseeds in a food processor and whizz for about 20 seconds. Add the banana, mango and soy milk and blend again for about 30 seconds until smooth. Serve straight away.

Nutrients (per serving)

Calories 340   Protein 10.5g (11%)

Total fat / saturated fat / omega-3 16.7g (41%) / 1.8g / 5.1g

Total carbs / sugar / fibre 42.6g (48%) / 25.0g / 10.1g

Vitamins and minerals A, B vitamins, C, calcium, copper, magnesium

---

Omega-3 Nut Butter

VG, VE, DF, GF

If you've never made your own nut butter, you'll be amazed at this little piece of kitchen alchemy. You have to blitz it in the food processor for at least ten minutes, but it slowly transforms from a nutty crumble to a lovely smooth butter. This version doubles as a kind of whole-food omega-3 supplement thanks to the walnuts, chia seeds and flaxseeds.

Prep: 15 mins   Cooking: 0 mins   Portions: 25 × 1 tablespoon

150g walnuts
150g almonds
15g ground flaxseeds (use pre-ground flaxseeds or grind them in a coffee grinder)

25g sunflower seeds
15g chia seeds
1 teaspoon salt
3 tablespoons neutral oil (I recommend organic rapeseed oil)

Place all the ingredients, except the oil, in a food processor. Process on low for 1 minute, adding the oil slowly, then increase the speed to as high as it will go and continue to process for approximately 10 minutes, or until the texture is smooth and butter-like. You may have to stop the machine a couple of times to scrape down the sides. Store in an airtight container in the fridge for 2–3 weeks.

Nutrients (per serving)

Calories 94   *Protein* 2.4g (9%)

Total fat / saturated fat / omega-3 18.9g (80%) / 9.7g / 0.9g

Total carbs / sugar / fibre 2.6g (11%) / 0.4g / 1.5g

Vitamins and minerals B1, B2, E, copper, magnesium, manganese

---

Hot Chia Porridge

VE, GF

If you don't like gloopy things, then this isn't for you, but I LOVE it and this simple recipe is absolutely heaving with omega-3 fatty acids and calcium. It's a welcome alternative to regular porridge, and you can pimp it in the same way by adding your favourite nuts, seeds and fruits.

Prep: 5 mins   Cooking: 10 mins   Serves: 1

250ml semi-skimmed milk (use non-dairy milk to make a
    VG/DF version)
3 tablespoons chia seeds
1 tablespoon date syrup
½ teaspoon ground cinnamon
½ teaspoon vanilla extract
1 small banana, sliced

Place the milk, chia seeds, date syrup, cinnamon and vanilla in a small saucepan over a medium heat and bring to the boil. Reduce the heat to low and simmer for 10 minutes, or until the mixture has thickened to a porridge-like consistency, stirring occasionally. Top with the sliced banana and serve.

Nutrients (per serving)

Calories 335   *Protein* 11.7g (14%)

Total fat / saturated fat / omega-3 9.9g (25%) / 3.7g / 2.7g

Total carbs / sugar / fibre 54.8 (61%) / 39.5g / 8.0g

Vitamins and minerals B2, B12, D, calcium, magnesium,
    phosphorus

Kedgeree Soup

—

I absolutely love smoked fish in all its forms, so kedgeree is a favourite brunch dish of mine. It occurred to me that it would work very well in soup form, and so I devised this: a hearty, comforting soup brimming with good fats and protein.

Prep: 5 mins   Cooking: 25 mins   Serves: 2 generously

2 eggs
250ml semi-skimmed milk
2 bay leaves
250g skinless and boneless smoked haddock fillets
1 teaspoon light olive oil
1 small onion, finely diced
500ml vegetable stock from a cube
1 teaspoon ground coriander
½ teaspoon ground turmeric
2 teaspoons medium curry powder
1 tablespoon plain flour (omit, to make this GF)
250g pre-cooked wholegrain rice (use a pouch if you like)
salt and freshly ground black pepper
handful of chopped flat-leaf parsley leaves (stalks removed)

Put the eggs in a medium-sized saucepan and cover with water. Bring to the boil on a high heat and then turn down the heat and simmer for 10 minutes until hard-boiled.

Meanwhile, pour the milk into a frying pan large enough to hold the fish. Place over a medium heat and add the bay leaves. When the milk is almost boiling, add the smoked haddock fillets. Reduce the heat to low and simmer for 10 minutes.

Meanwhile, heat the oil in a large saucepan over a low heat.

Add the onions and fry for 5 minutes until soft, adding a few tablespoons of the stock if it starts to stick. Increase the heat a little and add the coriander, turmeric and curry powder. Fry for 1 minute more, then add the flour and the rice and stir to coat before adding the stock. Add a good pinch of salt and pepper and simmer for 10 minutes.

Once the fish has poached in the milk, remove it to a plate and flake the fish, reserving the milk. Run the hard-boiled eggs under cold water, then peel and slice.

Now add the milk and flaked fish to the soup and simmer for a further 5 minutes. Serve with sliced boiled eggs arranged on top, and sprinkled with chopped parsley.

Nutrients (per serving)

Calories 490   *Protein* 46.4g (39%)

Total fat / saturated fat / omega-3 12.1g (22%) / 3.9g / 0.4g

Total carbs / sugar / fibre 47.7g (39%) / 10.0g / 5.3g

Vitamins and minerals B3, B6, B12, magnesium, phosphorus, selenium

---

Fabulous Feta Bake

VE, GF

Baking feta in the oven has been quite the craze for a while, so I may be a bit slow off the mark here – but better late than never! This dish is not a looker, I warn you, but I cannot emphasise enough how delicious it is. I'd serve it with a lovely crisp green salad, and perhaps some toasted sourdough.

Prep: 5 mins   Cooking: 25 mins   Serves: 4

> 250g cherry tomatoes
> 100g green olives (the type with the stones still in)
> 2 tablespoons extra virgin olive oil
> 1 tablespoon dried oregano
> salt and freshly ground black pepper
> 100g feta
> 400g tin chickpeas, drained and rinsed
> 150g spinach leaves
> juice of ½ lemon
> 1 tablespoon honey

Preheat the oven to 200°C/gas mark 7.

Place the tomatoes and olives in a large glass baking dish. Drizzle over the olive oil, sprinkle over the oregano, season well with salt and pepper, and stir everything together to coat. Place the chunk of feta in the middle (turning it over a couple of times to coat with the herby oil), then place in the oven for 20 minutes to bake.

Remove from the oven and add the chickpeas and spinach. Stir everything together roughly, then return to the oven for a further 5 minutes.

Meanwhile, combine the lemon juice and honey in a bowl.

Once the spinach is wilted down, remove the dish from the oven, mix everything together once more and drizzle over the honey and lemon before serving.

> **Nutrients (per serving)**
>
> *Calories* 277   *Protein* 9.8g (13%)
>
> *Total fat / saturated fat / omega-3* 16.8g (52%) / 5.2g / 0.2g
>
> *Total carbs / sugar / fibre* 25.2g (35%) / 9.2g / 6.7g
>
> *Vitamins and minerals* B9, C, K, calcium, magnesium, manganese

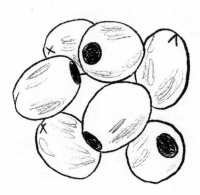

Griddled Figs with Rosemary, Honey, Feta and Toasted Walnuts

VE, GF

This is either a really classy snack or a sumptuous dinner-party starter; either way, it's absolutely delicious and unbelievable served with some seedy crackers (if you are feeling really adventurous, try making your own – see page 244). This recipe delivers plenty of omega-3, fibre and calcium, while feeling like a really decadent treat.

Prep: 5 mins   Cooking: 10 mins   Serves: 2

10g walnuts, chopped
1 tablespoon extra virgin olive oil
4 figs, halved
2 sprigs of rosemary
1 tablespoon honey
75g feta
freshly ground black pepper

Heat a large griddle pan (or frying pan, if you don't have one) over a medium heat and add the chopped walnuts. Toast until golden, tossing occasionally. Remove the walnuts from the pan and set aside on a plate.

Add the oil to the pan, followed by the figs, placing them cut-side down. Place the rosemary sprigs between the figs and drizzle over the honey. Allow to cook for approximately 3–4 minutes until the figs are softened and starting to brown, but watch the heat to make sure it doesn't burn; you want nice lines across the bottoms.

To serve, arrange the figs griddled-side up on a serving plate, then drizzle over the pan juices. Crumble over the feta, add a grind of black pepper and sprinkle over the toasted walnuts.

> **Nutrients (per serving)**
>
> *Calories* 299   *Protein* 6.9g (9%)
>
> *Total fat / saturated fat / omega-3* 18.4g (54%) / 6.9g / 0.6g
>
> *Total carbs / sugar / fibre* 30.1 (37%) / 26.6g / 3.4g
>
> *Vitamins and minerals* B2, B6, B12, calcium, phosphorus, zinc

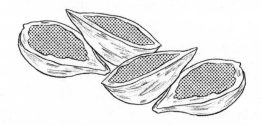

Roast Sardines with a Fennel and Dill Salad

DF, GF

Look for Cornish sardines on the fish counter at the supermarket or at a fishmonger if you have one nearby. If you can't find them, use mackerel instead. I love sardines simply roasted in the oven with oil, salt, pepper and lemon juice squeezed over. Here, I've served them with a lovely fresh fennel salad. To balance it up carbs-wise, you can have a few mini boiled potatoes on the side; there's lots of fibre in the skins.

Prep: 10 mins   Cooking: 15 mins   Serves: 4

1kg fresh sardines (2–3 per person, depending on the size)
1 tablespoon extra virgin olive oil
salt and freshly ground black pepper
1 lemon, quartered

For the salad
1 large fennel bulb (250g), trimmed and finely sliced
    (you can do this in a food processor)
100g watercress, washed thoroughly
10g dill, chopped

For the dressing
1 teaspoon Dijon mustard
1 tablespoon apple cider vinegar
1 tablespoon extra virgin olive oil
1 teaspoon honey
salt and freshly ground black pepper

Preheat the oven to 240°C/gas mark 10.

Place the sardines in a large baking dish. Drizzle over the extra virgin olive oil, add a sprinkle of salt and a grind of black pepper, and give everything a good toss. Space out the fish in the dish and put it in the middle of the oven to roast; this will only take 10–15 minutes.

Meanwhile, make the salad. Place the fennel, watercress and dill in a large salad bowl. In a small jug or bowl, whisk together the dressing ingredients, or shake them up in an airtight container. Dress the salad and divide between four plates. Place the grilled sardines on top and serve with lemon wedges for squeezing.

Nutrients (per serving)

Calories 528   *Protein* 41.0g (33%)

Total fat / saturated fat / omega-3 36.5g (62%) / 7.9g / 5.7g

Total carbs / sugar / fibre 7.4g (5%) / 4.1g / 2.2g

Vitamins and minerals B3, B12, D, iodine, magnesium, phosphorus, selenium

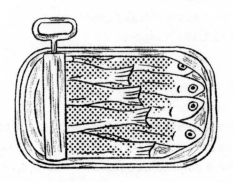

Baked Salmon with Tangy Kiwi Salsa

DF, GF

A simple salmon supper is something we all need up our sleeves, but just a quick word on sustainability. Look for the ASC mark for farmed salmon or the MSC mark for wild salmon, to make sure it has been fished responsibly. Here, the salmon is simply baked in parchment to keep it tender and delicious (and less messy!). The tangy salsa brings the whole thing to life.

Prep: 15 mins   Cooking: 10 mins   Serves: 4

4 × 130g salmon fillets
salt and freshly ground black pepper

For the salsa
2 kiwi fruits, peeled and diced
1 small red onion, finely diced
1 yellow pepper, finely diced
2 tomatoes, finely diced
1 garlic clove, finely grated
large handful of coriander (30g), finely chopped
1 tablespoon extra virgin olive oil
juice of 1 lime

Preheat the oven to 200°C/gas mark 7.

Season the salmon fillets and place on a large piece of baking parchment. Fold the ends of the parchment together and tuck underneath to make a parcel. Place this on a baking tray, then transfer to the oven and bake for 10 minutes.

Meanwhile, make the salsa. If you are short of time, you can roughly prepare all the ingredients, then whizz in a food processor for 10 seconds. If you prefer a chunkier salsa, then chop the vegetables by hand and place them all in a large bowl, then add the olive oil and lime juice. Season with salt and pepper and mix well.

Serve the fish with a good dollop of salsa over the top.

Nutrients (per serving)
Calories 318   *Protein* 28.0g (37%)
Total fat / saturated fat / omega-3 17.8g (50%) / 4.0g / 3.3g
Total carbs / sugar / fibre 11.4g (13%) / 5.5g / 2.2g
Vitamins and minerals This contains some of all the major
    vitamins, notably vitamin D, copper, phosphorus,
    selenium

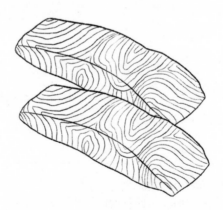

FIBRE-RICH

Fibre-rich Muesli

VG, VE, DF

Many shop-bought mueslis are high in sugar, so make this fibre-packed version instead. This uses psyllium husk, which is worth seeking out because it has an incredible 70g fibre per 100g. It is available in some supermarkets these days, and you can certainly get it in health-food shops or order it online. Serve with the milk of your choice – or Greek yogurt or kefir for maximum gut-health benefits – and top with grated apple or fresh raspberries for even more fabulous fibre.

Prep: 5 mins   Cooking: 0 mins   Portions: 10 × 55g

300g rolled oats
100g psyllium husk
50g flaked almonds

50g mixed seeds
50g raisins

Mix all the ingredients together and store in an airtight container. Will keep for 3 to 4 weeks.

Nutrients (per serving)
Calories 215   *Protein* 6.2g (13%)
Total fat / saturated fat / omega-3 7.1g (30%) / 0.7g / 0.2g
Total carbs / sugar / fibre 34.6g (57%) / 3.6g / 11.8g
Vitamins and minerals B1, B6, E, magnesium, manganese, zinc

Lentil Shakshouka

VE, GF

It's amazing how something simple, like adding a tin of lentils to a classic recipe, can up the nutritional ante. This riff on shakshouka delivers half your fibre needs for the day, has fabulous balanced macros and contains a whole host of micronutrients. I haven't included this in the recipe, but you can serve this sprinkled with chopped green herbs, like mint or parsley, if you happen to have some.

Prep: 10 mins   Cooking: 30 mins   Serves: 2 generously

1 tablespoon light olive oil
1 small red onion, finely sliced
1 garlic clove, finely grated
1 red pepper, deseeded and chopped
400g tin chopped tomatoes
400g tin lentils, drained and rinsed
1 teaspoon ground cumin
1 teaspoon paprika
½ teaspoon dried red chilli flakes
½ teaspoon light brown sugar
squeeze of lemon juice
4 eggs
salt and freshly ground black pepper
50g feta

Heat the oil in a medium-sized frying pan over a low heat. Add the onion and sauté for a few minutes until it begins to soften, then add the garlic and continue to sauté for another 2 minutes. Add the red pepper and cook for a further 5 minutes until softened.

The Recipes

Stir in the chopped tomatoes and lentils, along with the spices, sugar, lemon juice and 100ml water. Simmer together for 5 minutes. Make 4 evenly spaced wells in the tomato mixture and then crack one egg into each. Season well with salt and pepper and cover the pan with a lid. Cook for 10 minutes, or until the egg whites are firm but the yolks still runny. Once cooked, crumble over the feta and serve.

Nutrients (per serving)
Calories 418   *Protein* 26.7g (25%)
Total fat / saturated fat / omega-3 17.5g (37%) / 7.0g / 0.3g
Total carbs / sugar / fibre 41.2g (38%) / 15.8g / 14.8g
Vitamins and minerals A, B1, C, over 25% RNI of all
key minerals

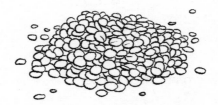

Courgette, White Bean and Parmesan Soup

GF

My soup-making has been transformed since I began to understand more about nutritional balance, and it's rare these days that I don't add some form of lean protein (like the beans here) and some healthy fat (like olive oil) rather than just veggies and stock. Although this packs a hefty 10.2g of fibre, it could just as easily be in the Vitamins and Minerals recipe section, as it contains such a huge range.

Prep: 10 mins   Cooking: 15 mins   Serves: 2 (generously)

1 tablespoon light olive oil
1 large leek (150g), trimmed and finely sliced
1 litre (1¾ pints) vegetable stock from 2 cubes
2 large courgettes (450g), grated
400g tin cannellini beans, drained and rinsed
juice of ½ lemon
handful of flat-leaf parsley, finely chopped
50g Parmesan, grated
salt and freshly ground black pepper

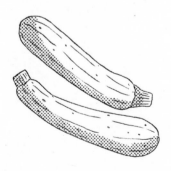

The Recipes

Heat the oil in a large saucepan over a medium heat. Add the leeks and sauté for 5 minutes to soften, adding a splash of the stock if the pan gets too dry. Next, add the stock, courgettes and beans and reduce the heat to low. Simmer for 15 minutes.

Add the lemon juice, parsley and Parmesan and stir well. Taste and season generously with salt and pepper. If you prefer a smooth soup, then go ahead and blend before serving.

Nutrients (per serving)

Calories 398   *Protein* 25.0g (21%)

Total fat / saturated fat / omega-3 11.8g (26%) / 4.7g / 0.2g

Total carbs / sugar / fibre 53.8g (53%) / 4.7g / 10.2g

Vitamins and minerals A, C, K, provides over 25% of the
   RNI of all the key minerals

Tuna and Wholemeal Fusilli Fagioli

DF

OK, so this is really just a posh name for a tuna pasta salad, but this store-cupboard superstar deserves to be a lunchtime regular. The trick here is to keep the pasta *al dente*; undercook it just a tad to avoid a soggy disaster. Popping a poached or fried egg on top is a nice twist on this classic.

Prep: 10 mins   Cooking: 10 mins   Serves: 2

100g dried wholemeal fusilli pasta
400g tin mixed beans, drained and rinsed
145g tin tuna in brine, drained
½ red onion, finely sliced
1 large tomato, roughly chopped
50g mixed pitted olives, roughly chopped
small handful of flat-leaf parsley leaves, chopped, to serve

For the dressing
1 tablespoon extra virgin olive oil
2 tablespoons apple cider vinegar
1 teaspoon Dijon mustard
1 teaspoon honey
½ teaspoon mixed dried herbs
a pinch each of salt and freshly ground black pepper

Cook the pasta according to the packet instructions, ensuring it is *al dente* and not over-cooked. Drain and rinse with cold water, then drain again and set aside.

In a large glass bowl, mix together the beans, tuna, red onion, tomato, olives and cold pasta.

In a separate bowl or jug, mix together the dressing ingredients, or shake them together in a lidded jar. Pour the dressing over the salad and toss gently to distribute. Sprinkle over the parsley and serve.

Nutrients (per serving)

Calories 450   *Protein* 29.8g (25%)

Total fat / saturated fat / omega-3 9.1g (18%) / 1.4g / 0.3g

Total carbs / sugar / fibre 67.0 (57%) / 6.5g / 11.0g

Vitamins and minerals B3, B6, B12, iodine, magnesium,
    manganese, selenium

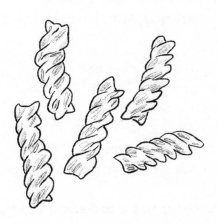

Everyday Dal

VG, VE, DF, GF

First of all, let me say I've played fast and loose with authenticity here in the interests of speed, but the main flavour elements are all there. This is about as simple a weekday meal as you'll get that still hits home nutritionally, and it provides a very welcome 10.6g fibre per serving. For even more, pair with toasted wholegrain pitas.

Prep: 10 mins   Cooking: 45 mins   Serves: 2 generously

1 tablespoon neutral oil
1 medium onion (100g), finely diced
2 garlic cloves, crushed
2–3cm piece of fresh root ginger, peeled and finely grated
1 teaspoon garam masala
1 teaspoon ground cumin
½ teaspoon cayenne pepper
100g dried red lentils
400g tin chopped tomatoes
500ml vegetable stock from a cube
salt
handful of chopped coriander leaves (optional)

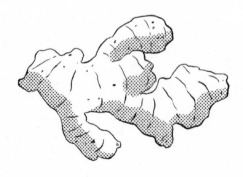

Heat the oil in a large saucepan over a medium heat. Add the onion and gently sauté for 5 minutes, then add the garlic, ginger, garam masala, cumin and cayenne pepper and mix well before adding the lentils. Cook for a few more minutes until everything is well combined. Add the tomatoes and stock and a good pinch of salt. Bring to the boil, then reduce the heat to low and loosely cover the pan with a lid. Simmer for 30–40 minutes, stirring occasionally. Add a little more water if it's getting too thick; it should eventually resemble a thick soup.

If you happen to have some fresh coriander, sprinkle some chopped leaves over the top to serve.

Nutrients (per serving)

Calories 317   *Protein* 15.1g (16%)

Total fat / saturated fat / omega-3 9.3g (25%) / 1.5g / 0.5g

Total carbs / sugar / fibre 47.5g (59%) / 7.9g / 10.6g

Vitamins and minerals B1, B6, C, copper, iron, zinc

Creamy Bean and Mushroom Stew
VE, GF

A bowlful of this, and you've already bagged half your recommended daily amount of fibre; that's definitely something your microbiome will thank you for. This stew is packed full of flavour and it keeps well, so make a double batch and park the rest in the fridge for quick weekday lunches. I absolutely love it with a slice of fresh, brown sourdough bread: a match made in fibre heaven.

Prep: 15 mins   Cooking: 40 mins   Serves: 2 (generously)

1 tablespoon neutral oil
1 small onion, finely diced
1 medium carrot, finely diced
2 celery sticks, finely diced
2 garlic cloves, finely grated
150g chestnut mushrooms, washed and quartered
salt and freshly ground black pepper
400g tin mixed beans, drained and rinsed
3 tablespoons light crème fraîche
2 teaspoons wholegrain mustard
1 teaspoon mixed dried herbs
1 teaspoon apple cider vinegar
500ml vegetable stock from a cube
handful of flat-leaf parsley, chopped, to serve

Heat the oil in a large saucepan over a medium heat. Add the onion, carrot and celery, and gently sauté for 5 minutes. Add the garlic, mushrooms and a good pinch of salt and pepper, and continue to sauté for a further 5 minutes. Add the beans, crème fraîche, mustard, dried herbs and apple cider vinegar, along with 400ml of the stock, and mix well to combine. Bring the whole lot to the boil, then reduce the heat to low and simmer for 30 minutes, stirring occasionally.

Use the remaining 100ml of stock to loosen if it's getting too thick. Serve topped with the chopped flat-leaf parsley.

Nutrients (per serving)
Calories 377   *Protein* 18.9g (17%)
Total fat / saturated fat / omega-3 10.9g (25%) / 2.7g / 0.5g
Total carbs / sugar / fibre 54.7g (58%) / 8.2g / 15.0g
Vitamins and minerals A, B2, K, calcium, iron, magnesium

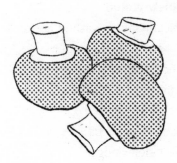

Smoky Black Bean, Aubergine and Red Pepper Tortillas

VG, VE, DF, GF (check the corn tortillas are fully GF)

Boy, oh boy, this packs a flavour punch, and I've yet to find a bean-avoider who doesn't like it! It's also got an incredible 16.5g of fibre per serving, which is over half your daily requirement. I serve it dolloped on hand-sized corn tortillas and topped with chopped avocado, tomato, Greek yogurt (not if you are dairy-free, obviously!) and chopped coriander. Deeelish.

Prep: 10 mins   Cooking: 40 mins   Serves: 4

1 tablespoon neutral oil
1 large red onion, finely diced
1 garlic clove, crushed
1 red pepper, finely diced
1 aubergine (250g), diced
2 teaspoons paprika
1 teaspoon hot chilli powder
salt
400g tin black beans, drained and rinsed
300ml vegetable stock from a cube

To serve
8 corn tortillas (the ones that are about the size of your hand)
1 avocado, peeled, stoned and diced
1 large ripe tomato, peeled and diced
handful of coriander leaves, chopped
1 teaspoon Greek yogurt per tortilla (omit, to make it VG/DF)

Heat the oil in a large saucepan over a medium heat. Add the onion and sauté for 3 minutes, then add the garlic and red pepper and continue to sauté for another 2 minutes. Add the aubergine, paprika, chilli powder and a large pinch of salt, and cook for a further 5 minutes, stirring to ensure the spices are well distributed throughout. Add the beans and stock and bring to the boil, then reduce the heat to low and simmer for 30 minutes, stirring occasionally. Almost all the liquid should reduce down so it resembles a vegetable chilli in consistency; add a drop of water if it's getting too dry.

To serve, take out four plates and place two corn tortillas on each plate. Divide the bean mixture between the tortillas, then top each one with tomato, avocado and chopped coriander, finishing with a blob of Greek yogurt, if using.

Nutrients (per serving)

Calories 372   *Protein* 13.3g (12%)

Total fat / saturated fat / omega-3 13.3g (30%) / 2.0g / 0.3g

Total carbs / sugar / fibre 54.8g (58%) / 8.9g / 16.5g

Vitamins and minerals B6, B9, C, copper, magnesium, phosphorus

---

Sweet Potato Falafel with Avocado and Tomato Salsa

VG, VE, DF

If you are a falafel fiend like me, then you'll know how important the crunchy exterior and soft, yielding centre are to their success – and these definitely deliver. A food processor will make this much quicker to make, and I like to bake my falafels rather than frying for a better texture. If you aren't GF or DF, serve in a wholemeal pita stuffed with the salsa and a spoonful of thick Greek yogurt.

Prep: 20 mins   Cooking: 40 mins   Serves: 4

100g fresh wholegrain breadcrumbs*
200g sweet potato, peeled and grated
150g carrots, peeled and grated
400g tin kidney beans, drained and rinsed
3 spring onions, finely sliced
2 teaspoons paprika
1 teaspoon hot chilli powder
1 teaspoon salt
½ teaspoon freshly ground black pepper
50g sesame seeds, for coating

For the salsa
1 ripe avocado, peeled, stoned and chopped
2 medium ripe tomatoes, diced
juice of ½ lemon
salt and freshly ground black pepper

If you are cooking these straight away, preheat the oven to 200°C/ gas mark 7 and line a baking tray with baking parchment.

* To make breadcrumbs, simply whizz up the bread in a food processor.

The Recipes

Place the grated vegetables in a large saucepan over a high heat and cover with water. Bring to the boil, then reduce the heat to low and simmer for 10 minutes. Drain well and transfer to the food processor.

Add the breadcrumbs, kidney beans, onions, spices, salt and pepper to the food processor as well, and whizz until all combined; you might have to stop and scrape down the sides once or twice.

Place the sesame seeds on a plate, then, taking small amounts of the mixture (approx. 30g each), form balls and roll them in the seeds. You can keep the balls in the fridge to cook later, or even freeze them at this stage.

To cook, place on the prepared tray and bake for 30 minutes.

When the falafels are almost ready, make the salsa. Combine all the ingredients in a bowl and serve straight away with the falafels; the salsa doesn't keep, as the avocado goes brown, so make it just before eating.

> **Nutrients (per serving)**
> *Calories* 355 *Protein* 12.2g (13%)
> *Total fat / saturated fat / omega-3* 17.0g (40%) / 2.6g / 0.2g
> *Total carbs / sugar / fibre* 43.4g (47%) / 8.8g / 13.4g
> *Vitamins and minerals* A, B6, K, magnesium, potassium, zinc

GUT HEALTH

Gut-friendly Smoothie

VE, GF

This smoothie is not only absolutely delicious, it also combines loads of goodies for your gut. It's a great entry-level use of kefir, a fermented yogurt that's teeming with beneficial bacteria, but which tastes quite sour on its own. Complete with figs, cherries, banana, nuts, seeds and honey, this smoothie is a very pleasant way to start the day and, as a side note, it has a good hit of omega-3, too.

Prep: 5 mins   Cooking: 0 mins   Serves: 1

- 5 almonds
- ½ tablespoon chia seeds
- 2 fresh figs, stalks removed, quartered
- 1 small banana, broken into pieces
- 75g frozen, unsweetened cherries
- 4 tablespoons plain kefir
- 1 teaspoon honey

Put the almonds in the blender first and whizz to grind up. Then add the remaining ingredients, along with 100ml water, and blend on high for 30 seconds until well combined. Enjoy straight away.

Nutrients (per serving)

Calories 280   *Protein* 7.5g (10%)

Total fat / saturated fat / omega-3 6.6g (20%) / 1.2g / 1.1g

Total carbs / sugar / fibre 53.7g (70%) / 38.4g / 8.2g

Vitamins and minerals A, B vitamins, C, calcium, magnesium, manganese

---

Ten-plant-foods Overnight Oats

VE, GF (use GF-certified oats)

Overnight oats are the easiest way to get a ton of gut goodies into your breakfast. I've designed this to include probiotics, in the form of kefir, and prebiotics, in the form of apples, oats and flaxseeds. A veritable good-bacteria bonanza, and a useful hit of omega-3 too.

Prep: 10 mins   Cooking: 0 mins   Serves: 3

100g rolled oats
1 tablespoon each chia seeds, flaxseeds, sunflower seeds and
    pumpkin seeds
1 tablespoon flaked almonds
5 walnut halves, chopped
5 dried apricots, chopped
1 small apple, grated, skin on
1 teaspoon ground cinnamon
150ml kefir, plus extra to serve if needed
200ml semi-skimmed milk, plus extra to serve if needed

Place all the ingredients in an airtight container and mix thoroughly. Put the lid on and pop in the fridge overnight. In the morning, give it a good mix, then place one serving in a bowl (this recipe makes three servings and will keep for three days). Add a little more kefir or milk to loosen if it needs it. As an option, top with fresh chopped fruit.

Nutrients (per serving)

Calories 361   *Protein* 14.6g (15%)

Total fat / saturated fat / omega-3 15.7g (36%) / 2.7g / 1.8g

Total carbs / sugar / fibre 44.5g (49%) / 15.1g / 9.0g

Vitamins and minerals B1, B2, E, magnesium, manganese, zinc

Good Guts Prebiotic Soup

VG, VE, DF

Prebiotics are a form of carbohydrate that the good bacteria in your gut love to feast on. This soup contains some of the best prebiotic foods out there, so your microbiota are in for a treat. This is best made using a food processor for speed and a better final texture. If you aren't DF, stir in a spoonful of Greek yogurt or kefir at the end for even more gut goodness.

Prep: 10 mins   Cooking: 30 mins   Serves: 4

1 onion, quartered
1 leek, trimmed and roughly chopped
1 tablespoon light olive oil
125g asparagus, woody ends removed, roughly chopped
1 courgette, trimmed and roughly chopped
800ml (scant 1½ pints) vegetable stock, made from 2 cubes
250g pouch of pre-cooked mixed grains
salt and freshly ground black pepper
juice of 1 lemon

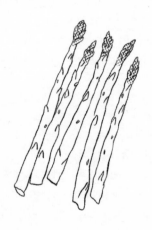

Using a food processor, finely chop the onion and leek.

Heat the oil in a large saucepan over a medium heat, then tip in the onion and leek and sauté gently while you chop the asparagus and courgette in the food processor, then add those to the pan as well.

Stir all the vegetables together and sauté for a further 2–3 minutes. Now add the stock and the grains. Stir well and season generously with salt and pepper.

Bring to the boil, then reduce the heat to low and simmer for 20 minutes.

Finally, add the lemon juice, stir well and taste. Add more salt and pepper if required before serving.

Nutrients (per serving)

Calories 171   *Protein* 4.9g (9%)

Total fat / saturated fat / omega-3 4.2g (21%) / 0.7g / 0.1g

Total carbs / sugar / fibre 31.0g (70%) / 5.1g / 6.3g

Vitamins and minerals A, B6, C, copper, manganese, selenium

Easy Kimchi

DF

If you have yet to dip your toe in the fermenting pond, then this is a good place to start. I learned how to make several fermented products when I was studying at Leith's, and this one was my favourite. I can't claim the recipe as my own, but it is one that I have adopted and think you will love it too. You can use it in the Kimchi and Spring Onion Omelette recipe on page 184.

Prep: 15 mins   Sitting time: 3 hours   Portions: 28 × 50g

280g carrots, thinly sliced
450g fennel, thinly sliced
400g Chinese leaf cabbage, chopped
75g golden caster sugar
1 tablespoon salt

For the paste
15g dried red chilli flakes
3 garlic cloves, finely grated
50g fresh root ginger, peeled and finely grated
4 teaspoons fish sauce
3 teaspoons light soy sauce (use tamari to make it GF)
5 spring onions, finely sliced

Sterilise a large, lidded storage jar with boiling water and allow it to dry thoroughly before you begin.

Place the carrot, fennel and cabbage in a large bowl. Add the sugar and salt and massage the vegetables with clean hands. Do this for at least 5 minutes until they start to release liquid. Cover with a tea towel and set aside for 2 hours.

In a small bowl, combine all the paste ingredients and mix well, then set aside.

After the 2 hours are up, add the paste to the vegetables and combine thoroughly. Pack the mixture into the storage jar, pressing down firmly. Be sure to pour the liquid remaining in the bowl into the jar. It needs to completely cover the vegetables, so top up with a little water if there's not enough. Leave 3cm of space at the top of the jar to allow the escaping fermenting gas some room. Leave the jar open at room temperature for 1 hour before closing the lid and putting in the fridge.

The kimchi can be eaten the next day, but the flavour will develop over the following weeks. It will keep for up to 6 months in the fridge.

Nutrients (per serving)

Calories 27   *Protein* 0.7g (7%)

Total fat / saturated fat / omega-3 0.2g (6%) / 0.0g / 0.0g

Total carbs / sugar / fibre 6.2g (87%) / 4.1g / 1.3g

Vitamins and minerals A, C, K, copper, manganese, potassium

Kimchi and Spring Onion Omelette

DF

This very simple recipe uses kimchi; you can buy this in the
supermarket or make your own (see page 182). Because it's whisked
in with the eggs, the kimchi delivers a very delicate, spicy Asian
twist rather than being overpowering. If you are already a kimchi
devotee, by all means add more to the mix, or simply dollop
another spoonful on top of the cooked omelette.

Prep: 2 mins   Cooking: 5 mins   Serves: 1

2 eggs
1 teaspoon neutral oil
2 tablespoons kimchi
1 spring onion, finely sliced
salt and freshly ground black pepper

Whisk together the eggs in a bowl, then add the kimchi and mix
well. Heat the oil in a large frying pan over a medium–high heat.
Add the egg mixture and swirl to cover the pan base. Add the
spring onion and season with salt and pepper. Cook for 3–4
minutes, then flip over and finish on the other side for a minute or
so. Eat immediately.

Nutrients (per serving)

Calories 196   *Protein* 13.6g (29%)

Total fat / saturated fat / omega-3 14.2g (65%) / 3.5g / 0.5g

Total carbs / sugar / fibre 3.0g (6%) / 1.2g / 0.7g

Vitamins and minerals B2, C, D, iron, phosphorus,
    selenium

Refreshing, Hydrating Salad

VE, DF, GF

I say salad, but this sits somewhere between a salad and salsa, and it's the perfect accompaniment to grilled fish. All the fruit and vegetables used have a high water content to help you stay hydrated and refreshed. This is best made a little in advance and kept in the fridge.

Prep: 15 mins   Cooking: 0 mins   Serves: 4 as a side dish

100g green grapes, halved
½ cucumber (150g), cut into 1cm cubes
1 small courgette (200g), cut into 2cm cubes
2 celery sticks, sliced
handful of fresh mint leaves, sliced

For the dressing
zest and juice of 1 lime
1 tablespoon extra virgin olive oil
1 teaspoon honey (use maple syrup to make it VG)
1 teaspoon apple cider vinegar
salt and freshly ground black pepper

Prepare the salad ingredients and place in a large bowl, then put in the fridge to chill. Combine the dressing ingredients in a small airtight container and give it a good shake to combine. Pour the dressing over the salad and toss well just before serving.

Nutrients (per serving)
Calories 79   Protein 2.2g (7%)
Total fat / saturated fat / omega-3 3.8g (42%) / 0.6g / 0.0g
Total carbs / sugar / fibre 11.3g (51%) / 6.7g / 1.8g
Vitamins and minerals A, C, K, copper, magnesium

Sticky Miso Maple Aubergines
VG, VE, DF, GF

This dish has a distinctly Chinese vibe to it; it's quite spicy, so dial down the chilli flakes if you aren't so keen. The trick here is to make sure the aubergine is cooked for long enough to be fully soft and a little charred at the edges – you'll need patience. This is a perfect side dish for four people with chicken or pork, but is an equally satisfying meal on its own, served with brown rice and a fried egg on top.

Prep: 10 mins   Cooking: 25 mins   Serves: 4 as a side dish

1 large (350g) aubergine, cut into long batons
1 teaspoon cornflour
1 tablespoon and 1 teaspoon neutral oil
2 spring onions, finely sliced
2 garlic cloves, finely sliced
2–3 cm piece of fresh root ginger, peeled and finely diced
½ teaspoon dried red chilli flakes (or to taste)
2 teaspoons sesame seeds

For the sauce
2 tablespoons miso paste
1 tablespoon maple syrup
juice of 1 lime

Prepare the aubergine by cutting it in half lengthways, then cutting each half into three pieces, and then each third into 2cm-wide batons. Place the batons in a bowl and sprinkle over the cornflour, then toss well.

Combine all the sauce ingredients in a bowl along with 100ml water, and mix well with a fork.

Now heat the 1 tablespoon oil in a wok or large saucepan over a medium heat. Add the aubergine batons and sauté for around 15 minutes until they are softened and the edges are slightly browned. Keep an eye on them, stirring occasionally.

When the aubergine batons are tender, remove them from the pan and set aside on a plate. Add the remaining 1 teaspoon of oil to the pan, followed by the spring onions, garlic, ginger and chilli flakes, and fry for a minute or so. Return the aubergine to the pan and add the sauce mixture. Continue to cook for several minutes until the sauce has thickened.

Meanwhile, in a small non-stick frying pan, toast the sesame seeds for a few minutes until golden. When everything is ready, sprinkle the sesame seeds over the aubergine pieces to serve.

Nutrients (per serving)
Calories 93   *Protein* 2.5g (8%)
Total fat / saturated fat / omega-3 3.9g (36%) / 0.4g / 0.3g
Total carbs / sugar / fibre 13.9g (56%) / 7.1g / 3.7g
Vitamins and minerals B2, B6, K, copper, magnesium, manganese

Indonesian Vegetables and Tempeh in a Coconut Milk Broth

DF, GF

Although there's quite a long list of ingredients here, don't be put off: this dish is so simple to make and is a great introduction to tempeh, tofu's firmer, more approachable cousin. You can buy tempeh in any independent health-food shop, and it's widely available in supermarkets these days, too. Tempeh is basically fermented soy beans, so it's packed with probiotics. It's also a great source of plant-based lean protein and omega-3, and it contains a wide array of vitamins and minerals. For a VG/VE version, replace the fish sauce with lime juice.

Prep: 15 mins   Cooking: 20 mins   Serves: 4

400ml can light coconut milk
salt
200g block of tempeh, cut into 2cm cubes
1 carrot, peeled and thinly sliced
½ small white cabbage, sliced
200g mangetout
1 small aubergine, cut into chunks
1 lime, quartered

For the spice paste
1 stick lemongrass (outer layer taken off), roughly chopped
2 small red chillies, deseeded
1 small red onion, roughly chopped
3 garlic cloves, roughly chopped
2–3cm piece of fresh root ginger, peeled and roughly chopped
1 teaspoon ground cumin
1 teaspoon ground coriander

1 teaspoon ground turmeric
1 tablespoon fish sauce
2 tablespoons neutral oil

Place all the spice paste ingredients in a blender with 2 tablespoons water and blend for a minute or so until it forms a paste. If too thick to blend properly, add a drop more water.

Place a wok over a medium heat and fry the spice paste for 2–3 minutes, being careful not to let it burn. Add the coconut milk and an equal amount of water and mix well until fully combined with the spice paste. Taste and add salt as required. Add the tempeh and vegetables and bring up to just about boiling. Then reduce the heat to low, and let it simmer for 20 minutes. Serve with lime wedges for squeezing over.

Nutrients (per serving)

Calories 291   *Protein* 13.1g (15%)

Total fat / saturated fat / omega-3 19.3g (57%) / 8.0g / 0.5g

Total carbs / sugar / fibre 21.8g (28%) / 8.5g / 6.1g

Vitamins and minerals A, C, K, copper, iron, manganese

FIVE-A-DAY

Sunshine Smoothie

VG, VE, DF, GF (use GF-certified oats)

My aim with this recipe is to get a load of plant foods in early doors at breakfast. I counted 12 in my version, with the mixed seeds having four varieties included, so you are definitely feeding your microbiome here as well as getting plenty of vitamins and minerals.

Prep: 10 mins   Cooking: 0 mins   Serves: 1

- 1 teaspoon mixed seeds
- 4 almonds
- 2 walnut halves
- 1 tablespoon rolled oats
- 1 small banana (100g), peeled
- 100g frozen mango
- 1 teaspoon finely grated fresh root ginger
- juice of 1 orange
- squeeze of lemon juice
- 1 teaspoon maple syrup
- 5 ice cubes

Put the seeds, almonds, walnuts and oats in a food processor or blender and whizz on high for 20 seconds. Add the remaining ingredients, along with 100ml water, and blend on high for a minute or so until smooth and creamy. You may need to stop and scrape down the sides once or twice. Drink immediately.

Nutrients (per serving)

Calories 328   *Protein* 6.6g (7%)

Total fat / saturated fat / omega-3 8.7g (22%) / 0.9g / 0.5g

Total carbs / sugar / fibre 62.1g (71%) / 39.5g / 6.7g

Vitamins and minerals A, B6, C, E, copper, magnesium, manganese

---

Many Veg and Cheddar Soup

VE, GF

Soup is one of the best ways to pack in the veg, but the more vegetables you use, the more you risk it turning into a flavour confusion. I've picked eight everyday vegetables that work together brilliantly, with some grated Cheddar added to enrich the flavour. This soup is blended to a very smooth consistency, which puts me in mind of a French *'potage'* – never a bad thing.

Prep: 10 mins   Cooking: 25 mins   Serves: 4

1 onion, quartered
1 leek, trimmed
1 carrot, peeled and roughly chopped
1 celery stick, roughly chopped
1 tablespoon light olive oil
150g broccoli florets
150g cauliflower florets
40g red lentils
1 medium potato (200g), washed but skin left on
1 litre (1¾ pints) vegetable stock, made from 2 cubes
½ teaspoon salt
freshly ground black pepper
100g spinach
75g Cheddar, grated

Place the onion, leek, carrot and celery in a food processor and whizz until relatively finely chopped.

Heat the oil in a large saucepan over a medium heat and add the contents of the food processor. Mix well to begin to soften.

Now chop up the broccoli and cauliflower florets in the food processor until they look a bit like rice, then add to the pan, along with the red lentils, and mix well. Next, chop up the potato in the food processor, then add to the pan, along with the stock, salt and a good grinding of black pepper. Increase the heat to bring to the boil, then reduce the heat to low and simmer for 15 minutes.

Add the spinach leaves and simmer for a further 5 minutes. Now blend the soup. You can do this in the food processor, but you'll need to work in batches; if you do too much at once, it can spill out. You need to blend for a good minute or so to get the soup super smooth. I prefer to do this in two batches in a high-speed blender for the best texture.

Once blended, return to the pan (give the pan a rinse first to get rid of any bits), and reheat. Add the grated cheese, stir until melted in, then serve.

Nutrients (per serving)

Calories 226   *Protein* 11.6g (17%)

Total fat / saturated fat / omega-3 7.4g (30%) / 3.9g / 0.2g

Total carbs / sugar / fibre 30.9g (53%) / 5.8g / 6.3g

Vitamins and minerals A, B6, B9, C, K, provides at least
    15% RNI of all key minerals

Curtido (Mexican Slaw)

VG, VE, DF, GF

If you've never heard of *curtido*, then prepare to meet your new favourite side dish. It's best likened to a non-creamy coleslaw: super fresh and zingy and bursting with goodness. There is a little sugar – 2 teaspoons, to be precise – which is needed to balance out the vinegar, but as it serves four, that's only ½ teaspoon each.

Prep: 10 mins   Cooking: 2 mins   Serves: 4

1 small white cabbage (600g), finely sliced*
1 large red onion (150g), finely sliced*
2 large carrots (250g), grated*
100ml apple cider vinegar
2 teaspoons caster sugar
½ teaspoon salt
small handful of coriander leaves, roughly chopped (optional)

Place the shredded veg in a bowl. Heat the vinegar, sugar and salt in a small saucepan over a low heat for a couple of minutes until the sugar is dissolved. Pour over the vegetables and mix well. Chill in the fridge for at least 30 minutes before serving. The coriander leaves can be added just before serving.

Nutrients (per serving)
Calories 92   Protein 3.0g (9%)
Total fat / saturated fat / omega-3 0.4g (3%) / 0.1g / 0.1g
Total carbs / sugar / fibre 20.6g (88%) / 11.6g / 6.2g
Vitamins and minerals A, C, K, manganese

---

* To prepare the vegetables, it's easiest to simply use the finest slicing and grating attachments on your food processor.

Roasted Veg Greek Salad

VE, GF

Who doesn't love a Greek salad? I certainly do, and on a cold
winter's day, I suddenly had the idea for this roasted version.
It's a great way to pack in some veg and take an instant trip to
the Med from your kitchen table. It's lovely stuffed into a
wholemeal pita for lunch, or you could serve with some grilled
fish for dinner.

Prep: 10 mins   Cooking: 30 mins   Serves: 2

1 red pepper, cut into chunks
1 large courgette (200g), cut into 1 cm rounds
1 large red onion (150g), cut into chunks
1 tablespoon extra virgin olive oil
salt and freshly ground black pepper
200g cherry tomatoes
1 tablespoon red wine vinegar
1 teaspoon dried oregano
100g feta, broken into chunks

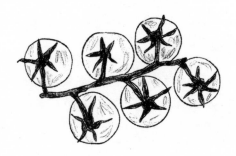

Preheat the oven to 200°C/gas mark 7.

Place the red pepper, courgette and onion in a large glass baking dish. Drizzle over the olive oil and season with salt and pepper. Toss to coat well, then roast for 20 minutes.

Remove from the oven, add the tomatoes and mix well. Place back in the oven for a further 10 minutes.

Remove from the oven and allow to cool for half an hour or so until at room temperature. Drizzle over the red wine vinegar and sprinkle over the oregano. Mix well, then place in a serving bowl and dot the feta chunks on top to serve.

Nutrients (per serving)

Calories 292   *Protein* 11.1g (14%)

Total fat / saturated fat / omega-3 18.3g (56%) / 8.6g / 0.3g

Total carbs / sugar / fibre 22.8g (30%) / 14.6g / 6.0g

Vitamins and minerals A, B6, C, calcium, phosphorus, zinc

Zingy, Grainy, Grated Salad

VE, DF, GF

If you've never made a grated salad before, all I can say is: you're welcome! This is the quickest way to get a load of plant foods on your plate, but you do need a food processor with a grater attachment, otherwise it's a bit of a faff. The joy of this is you can bung in any grate-able vegetables you happen to have to hand. I've featured my favourites here, and it's all pulled together with a lovely, tangy citrus dressing. You can swap the honey for maple syrup for a vegan version.

Prep: 10 mins   Cooking: 0 mins   Serves: 4

250g pouch of pre-cooked mixed grains*
1 small red cabbage (250g), cut into wedges
1 medium carrot (150g), peeled and halved
1 medium courgette (200g), trimmed and halved
1 red pepper, deseeded and quartered
handful of mint leaves, chopped, to serve

For the dressing
1 tablespoon extra virgin olive oil
2 tablespoons orange juice
1 tablespoon lemon juice
1 tablespoon apple cider vinegar
1 teaspoon lemon zest
1 teaspoon honey
pinch of salt

* *I use Merchant Gourmet's 'Glorious Grains' mix, but any pre-cooked grains, lentils or rice will work*

To refresh the grains, boil a kettle of water. Empty the pouch of grains into a sieve and, holding it over the sink, pour over the boiling water. Now run the cold tap over the grains and drain thoroughly.

Next, put all the vegetables through the food processor on the coarse grater setting, then place in a large salad bowl, add the grains and mix well.

Put all the dressing ingredients in a lidded jar and give it a good shake. Pour over the vegetables and grains and toss thoroughly using salad servers. Add the chopped mint leaves and mix through just before serving.

Nutrients (per serving)

Calories 209   *Protein* 8.0g (9%)

Total fat / saturated fat / omega-3 4.9g (21%) / 0.7g / 0.1g

Total carbs / sugar / fibre 37.4g (70%) / 8.4g / 6.5g

Vitamins and minerals A, B6, C, magnesium, manganese, zinc

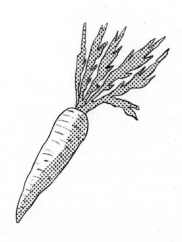

Asparagus and Pea Shoot Salad with Grapefruit and Soft Goat's Cheese

VE, GF

This is such a pretty salad. It's simple, too, but with a good range of vitamins and minerals, along with protein from the goat's cheese. I can picture it resplendent on a trestle table outside in the summer, the perfect accompaniment to some grilled fish. If you can't get pea shoots, some watercress or rocket leaves would also work well.

Prep: 10 mins   Cooking: 2 mins   Serves: 2

1 pink grapefruit
10g hazelnuts, chopped
100g asparagus tips
80g pea shoots
small handful of mint leaves, finely chopped
75g soft goat's cheese

For the dressing
1 tablespoon extra virgin olive oil
1 teaspoon apple cider vinegar
1 teaspoon Dijon mustard
salt and freshly ground black pepper

Prepare the grapefruit using a sharp knife in a shallow bowl so you can collect any juice that escapes. Slice off the top and bottom of the fruit, then, placing it down on one of the flat ends, pare off the skin, going around the fruit until it has all been removed. Now use the knife to slide down each segment to remove the pink flesh, leaving the membrane behind.

Transfer any juices to a lidded container, and add the dressing ingredients. Shake well to combine, then set aside.

Heat a small, non-stick frying pan over a medium heat and toast the chopped hazelnuts for a few minutes until golden.

Now blanch the asparagus by placing it in a heatproof bowl and pouring over boiled water from the kettle. Leave to sit for 2–3 minutes, then drain and run under cold water.

Assemble the salad by placing the pea shoots, asparagus and mint leaves in a large bowl. Pour over the dressing and toss well to coat. Place in a pretty serving bowl and arrange the grapefruit segments on top. Dot small amounts of goat's cheese around the salad, then sprinkle over the toasted hazelnuts. Eat immediately.

Nutrients (per serving)
Calories 262   *Protein* 10.9g (16%)
Total fat / saturated fat / omega-3 18.1g (60%) / 6.7g / 0.1g
Total carbs / sugar / fibre 17.4g (24%) / 9.8g / 4.2g
Vitamins and minerals A, B2, C, K, this contains a good
    amount of many of the essential minerals

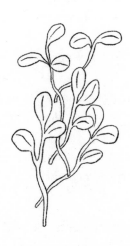

Garlic Greens

VG, VE, DF, GF

This is my go-to veggie side dish; I make it at least once a week. You can vary the vegetables, but I find that a mix of three varieties works best. Here, I've opted for asparagus, mangetout and green beans. The trick is to blanch the veg in boiling water first to make sure they retain their crunch and colour.

Prep: 5 mins   Cooking: 10 mins   Serves: 4

120g fine green beans, trimmed
100g asparagus tips, halved if very long
200g mangetout
1 teaspoon neutral oil
3 garlic cloves, finely chopped
200ml vegetable stock, made with 1 cube
pinch of salt (if needed)

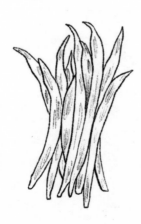

Bring a large wok or saucepan of water to the boil. Once on a rolling simmer, add the green beans. Blanch for 2 minutes, then remove and place in a large bowl of cold water. Now add the asparagus and mangetout to the pan of boiling water and blanch for 1 minute, before removing and placing in the cold water. Drain the vegetables.

Tip the water out of the wok and place it over a high heat. Add the oil, followed by the garlic. Fry for 20 seconds or so, then add the stock. Once the stock is really hot, add the vegetables. Stir-fry on high for 2–3 minutes. The vegetables should be vibrantly green and still quite crunchy. The stock will reduce down a bit, but you want some left as a kind of garlicky jus to pour over. Taste and season with salt if it needs it; this will depend on how salty your stock is. Serve straight away.

Nutrients (per serving)

Calories 53   *Protein* 2.8g (16%)

Total fat / saturated fat / omega-3 1.5g (24%) / 0.2g / 0.1g

Total carbs / sugar / fibre 8.2g (60%) / 3.6g / 2.7g

Vitamins and minerals A, C, K, copper, iron, manganese

Yellow Chicken Curry with Coconut and Cardamom

DF, GF

This is a light and aromatic chicken curry, packed with vegetables, with a gorgeous yellow colour that makes it a feast for the eyes as well as the tummy. As you'd expect with all that veg, there's a lot of vitamin C in here, as well as a whole host of essential minerals. A word on the heat: if you like a mild curry, use large green chillies here; if you like it hotter, use the smaller bird's eye ones. I think this goes best with brown basmati rice, as the sauce is not overly thick, so it needs something to run into.

Prep: 15 mins   Cooking: 30 mins   Serves: 4

1 tablespoon neutral oil
1 small onion, finely diced
2 garlic cloves, finely grated
2 fresh green chillies, deseeded and finely chopped
1 teaspoon ground cumin
1 teaspoon ground coriander
1 teaspoon ground turmeric
10 cardamom pods, gently crushed to open
1 teaspoon salt
450g mini chicken fillets
1 head cauliflower (400g), chopped into small florets
1 large courgette (350g), chopped into chunks
1 yellow pepper, deseeded and chopped into chunks
400ml can light coconut milk
500ml vegetable stock, made from 1 cube
juice of ½ lime
small handful of coriander leaves, chopped, to serve

The Recipes

Heat the oil in a large saucepan or wok over a medium heat. Add the onion and sauté gently for 5 minutes, then add the garlic, chillies, spices and salt. Stir well and cook for another minute or two, then add the chicken fillets and stir to coat with the spicy mixture. Add the vegetables and mix again, then stir in the coconut milk and stock. Increase the heat to high until the mixture is nearly boiling, then reduce to low and simmer for 30 minutes, stirring occasionally.

Just before serving, add the lime juice. Sprinkle over the coriander leaves to serve.

Nutrients (per serving)

Calories 338   *Protein* 36.7g (41%)

Total fat / saturated fat / omega-3 15.5g (40%) / 7.7g / 0.4g

Total carbs / sugar / fibre 17.4g (19%) / 5.9g / 4.6g

Vitamins and minerals B3, B6, C, iron, magnesium,
        potassium, zinc

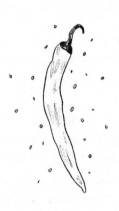

VITAMINS AND MINERALS

Glamour Fruits Yogurt Bowl

VE, GF

If you want to feel a bit special at breakfast time, then this is a very healthy way to do it. Glamour fruits are those with a bit of an exotic twist; my favourites are passion fruit, figs and pomegranate, so that's what I've included here.

Prep: 5 mins   Cooking: 0 mins   Serves: 1

100g Greek yogurt
1 teaspoon date syrup
1 fig, sliced
pulp of 1 passion fruit

handful of pomegranate seeds
1 tablespoon flaked almonds
1 tablespoon sunflower seeds
1 tablespoon rolled oats

Place the yogurt in a bowl and drizzle over the date syrup. Top with the sliced fig, passion fruit pulp and pomegranate seeds.

Heat a small frying pan over a medium–high heat and add the almonds, seeds and oats. Toast for a couple of minutes until golden, tossing occasionally. Sprinkle the toasted mixture over the fruit and serve.

Nutrients (per serving)

Calories 328   *Protein* 18.0g (21%)

Total fat / saturated fat / omega-3 13.7g (35%) / 1.3g / 0.0g

Total carbs / sugar / fibre 38.0g (44%) / 21.7g / 8.0g

Vitamins and minerals B2, B12, E, calcium, magnesium, zinc

Crab Guacamole Toast-topper

—

This recipe is inspired by one I found on the BBC Good Food website. The original was provided by Seafood and Eat It, who make delicious shellfish products and whose 'Fifty Fifty Crab' I recommend for this recipe. I've tweaked it slightly to really maximise the health benefits, but the main event here is that it's completely stuffed full of vitamin B12, with a good hit of most of the other micronutrients, too.

Prep: 10 mins   Cooking: 0 mins   Serves: Enough for 4 toasts

  100g pack mixed brown and white crabmeat
  ½ teaspoon mild curry powder
  1 tablespoon Greek yogurt
  1 tablespoon lime juice
  small handful of coriander leaves, finely chopped
  1 small ripe tomato, chopped
  ½ small red onion (40g), finely diced
  1 avocado, peeled, stoned and chopped
  salt and freshly ground black pepper
  1 teaspoon sesame seeds
  4 slices of seeded sourdough bread (or other wholegrain
     bread)

In a large bowl, combine the crab, curry powder, yogurt, lime juice, coriander, tomato and red onion.

In another bowl, mash the avocado with a fork, then add this to the crab mixture and stir together. Taste and season with salt and pepper.

Heat a small, non-stick frying pan over a medium–high heat and add the sesame seeds. Fry for a few minutes, tossing occasionally until golden.

Toast the bread, then divide the crab mixture between the toasts. Top with the sesame seeds and serve.

Nutrients (per serving)

Calories 251   *Protein* 16.1g (26%)

Total fat / saturated fat / omega-3 10.3g (35%) / 1.7g / 0.4g

Total carbs / sugar / fibre 25.3g (39%) / 4.2g / 7.2g

Vitamins and minerals A, B12 (and the other B vitamins), C, E, K, also contains some of all the major minerals

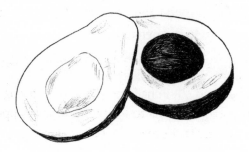

Healthy Potato Salad

VE, GF

I wanted to include this recipe because not a lot of people know that your common or garden potato is a really good source of vitamin C. In fact, a serving of this salad contains more than a third of your daily dose. I've created this healthier version by subbing in Greek yogurt for mayo, which is gut-friendly and lower-calorie – as well as being tangy and delicious, of course.

Prep: 5 mins   Cooking: 10 mins   Serves: 4

500g mini potatoes
salt and freshly ground black
   pepper
4 tablespoons thick Greek
   yogurt

1 teaspoon Dijon mustard
squeeze of lemon juice
2 spring onions, finely sliced
small handful of chives,
   chopped (optional)

Place the mini potatoes, with their skins on, in a saucepan of salted boiling water. Bring to the boil and boil for 10 minutes, or until tender. Drain and place in cold water.

Mix together the remaining ingredients in a bowl and season well.

Drain the potatoes, then cut in half and place in a serving bowl. Add the yogurt mixture and toss well to fully coat. If you happen to have some chives you can scatter some over before serving.

Nutrients (per serving)

Calories 109   *Protein* 3.2g (9%)

Total fat / saturated fat / omega-3 6.7g (5%) / 0.4g / 0.0g

Total carbs / sugar / fibre 23.1g (86%) / 1.9g / 3.0g

Vitamins and minerals B6, C, K, copper, phosphorus,
   potassium

Kale, Halloumi and Tomato Salad with a Caper Lemon Dressing

VE, GF

This tasty salad was an instant hit with my recipe-testers, and it's a great way to get most of your daily calcium and vitamin C needs in one go. Halloumi is a winner any day of the week, and although initially I wasn't so keen on kale (a bit chewy!), once I learned the trick of softening it by gently massaging it with olive oil, I was converted. I hope you agree that this is an excellent way to get some of your daily vitamins.

Prep: 10 mins   Cooking: 15 mins   Serves: 4

200g kale
1 tablespoon extra virgin olive oil
20 cherry tomatoes
250g halloumi cheese, cut into 1cm slices

For the dressing
1 tablespoon extra virgin olive oil
2 tablespoons apple cider vinegar
juice of 1 lemon
1 garlic clove, finely grated
1 teaspoon wholegrain mustard
1 teaspoon honey
1 teaspoon capers, drained

Place the kale in a large bowl. Pour over the extra virgin olive oil and gently massage for a minute or so until the leaves soften. Set aside.

With your hands still greasy, pick up the cherry tomatoes and gently handle until they are lightly coated with oil, then place them in a non-stick frying pan over a medium–high heat. Pan-fry for 5 minutes or so, rolling the tomatoes around the pan from time to time so each side gets slightly cooked. Remove the tomatoes from the pan and set aside in a bowl, then place the halloumi slices in the pan, turning after 2–3 minutes (or when golden) to brown on each side. Remove from the pan.

In a small bowl or jug, combine all the dressing ingredients and mix well.

Arrange the kale in a large serving bowl, then top with the halloumi and tomatoes and drizzle over the dressing. Serve immediately.

Nutrients (per serving)

Calories 260   *Protein* 11.2g (17%)

Total fat / saturated fat / omega-3 20.6g (70%) / 10.3g / 0.3g

Total carbs / sugar / fibre 9.6g (13%) / 5.5g / 1.9g

Vitamins and minerals A, C, K, calcium

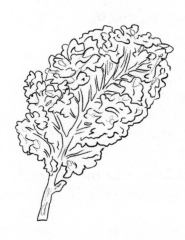

Nutrify Salad

VE, GF

The easiest way to get iron into your diet is by eating red meat, but for both health and ethical reasons, many of us are trying to reduce our meat consumption. Thankfully, there are lots of plant-based sources of iron, which I've combined in this nutrifying salad, along with plenty of vitamin C to help the iron be absorbed. It also delivers over 25% of the RNI of a host of other nutrients, including calcium, vitamin E, magnesium and zinc. My lovely recipe-tester Marie pointed out that this recipe uses half a tin of chickpeas and half a lemon, which is a bit annoying, so you can either double the quantities to serve 4, or perhaps make a little lemony hummus!

Prep: 10 mins   Cooking: 3 mins   Serves: 2

2 tablespoons pumpkin seeds
115g baby spinach
½ 400g tin chickpeas, drained and rinsed
40g dried apricots, finely sliced
100g cherry tomatoes, quartered
40g black kalamata olives, halved
40g feta, crumbled

For the dressing
1 tablespoon extra virgin olive oil
juice and zest of ½ lemon
1 teaspoon honey
1 teaspoon dried thyme
salt and freshly ground black pepper

Place a small, non-stick frying pan over a medium heat and toast the pumpkin seeds for 2–3 minutes, tossing a few times in the pan.

Put all the dressing ingredients in a small, lidded container and shake well to combine.

Place the spinach leaves in a large serving bowl, then add the chickpeas, apricots, tomatoes and olives. Pour over the dressing and toss well to coat everything thoroughly. Finally, crumble over the feta and sprinkle over the toasted pumpkin seeds to serve.

Nutrients (per serving)

Calories 344   *Protein* 12.3g (13%)

Total fat / saturated fat / omega-3 18.5g (46%) / 5.0g / 0.2g

Total carbs / sugar / fibre 37.5g (41%) / 18.8g / 8.4g

Vitamins and minerals A, C, E, K, calcium, iron, magnesium, zinc

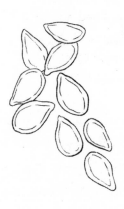

Pan-fried Rainbow Trout with Mushrooms and Chard

GF

Rainbow trout is a fabulous sustainable alternative to salmon, and contains almost a third of the fat, at just 135 calories per 100g. It's a good source of vitamin D, too, as are mushrooms, the only plant-food source of this critical vitamin. I love this dish served with some wild rice to balance up the macros.

Prep: 15 mins   Cooking: 15 mins   Serves: 4

4 × 130g rainbow trout fillets
salt and freshly ground black pepper
2 tablespoons salted butter
300g button mushrooms, sliced
3 garlic cloves, finely grated
2 tablespoons apple cider vinegar
200g Swiss chard, roughly chopped
20g flat-leaf parsley, roughly chopped
1 tablespoon neutral oil
1 lemon, cut into 4 wedges

Pat dry the fish fillets with kitchen paper, then season well on both sides with salt and pepper and set aside.

Melt the butter in a large saucepan or wok (choose one with a lid) over a medium heat. Add the mushrooms and season well with salt and pepper. Sauté, stirring occasionally, for 5 minutes until nicely browned. Now add the garlic and sauté for a further 2 minutes, then add the vinegar and 4 tablespoons water. Mix well, then add the chard and parsley. Reduce the heat to low and pop on the lid. It will take about 10 minutes for the chard to wilt down; be sure to stir from time to time.

Meanwhile, heat a large, non-stick frying pan over a medium heat. Add the oil and swirl around to coat the base of the pan. Place the fish fillets in the pan, skin-side down, and leave to cook until the skin is crispy. This will take around 10 minutes. If the pan has a lid, then cover it loosely just to avoid the fat spattering everywhere. Once the skin is done, flip the fillets over for just a minute to cook the other side.

Divide the mushroom and chard mixture between four plates and arrange a fillet of fish on top of each. Serve with lemon wedges, for squeezing.

Nutrients (per serving)

Calories 310   *Protein* 30.6g (40%)

Total fat / saturated fat / omega-3 18.3g (53%) / 5.4g / 1.7g

Total carbs / sugar / fibre 6.5g (7%) / 2.4g / 1.9g

Vitamins and minerals B12, D, K, magnesium, selenium, zinc

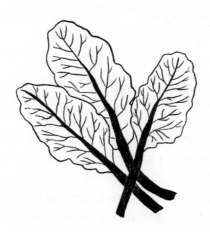

Healthy Palak Paneer
VE, GF

Paneer is a kind of white cheese, a bit like a softer halloumi. It is widely used in Indian cooking and you can find it in all the big supermarkets. This is a delicious, mild spinach curry. The paneer serves to add texture and protein to the dish, and it's packed with vitamins and minerals to boot. Serve over some brown basmati rice, or toast some wholemeal pitas to dip into the gorgeous green sauce.

Prep: 10 mins   Cooking: 20 mins   Serves: 4

1 tablespoon neutral oil
350g paneer, cut into 2cm cubes
1 small red onion, finely diced
2 garlic cloves, finely grated
1 tablespoon finely grated fresh root ginger
1 teaspoon chilli powder
1 teaspoon garam masala
2 teaspoons ground cumin
2 teaspoons ground coriander
1 tablespoon tomato purée
1 ripe tomato, diced
350g frozen spinach (defrosted)
120g plain yogurt
salt and freshly ground black pepper
squeeze of lemon juice

Heat the oil in a large, non-stick frying pan over a medium heat. Add the paneer cubes and gently brown all over – it takes about a minute on each side. Remove the paneer from the pan and set aside in a bowl.

Now add the onion, garlic and ginger to the same pan and sauté gently for 2 minutes, then add the chilli powder, garam masala, cumin and coriander and stir together. Add the tomato purée and mix until well combined, then add the diced tomato and let it all cook together for a further minute. Stir in the spinach and 300ml water, then let it simmer for about 5 minutes.

Remove the pan from the heat and pour the contents into a blender. Add the yogurt and blend on high for 30 seconds or so, until the mixture resembles a green smoothie. Return it to the pan, taste and season really well with salt and pepper. Add a good squeeze of lemon juice to freshen, then return the browned paneer cubes to the pan and reheat before serving.

Nutrients (per serving)

Calories 366   *Protein* 21.8g (22%)

Total fat / saturated fat / omega-3 25.8g (63%) / 12.2g / 0.5g

Total carbs / sugar / fibre 14.5g (15%) / 7.1g / 4.2g

Vitamins and minerals A, B12, K, calcium, magnesium, zinc

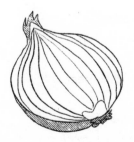

Simple Lamb and Chickpea Tagine
DF, GF

One of my favourite recipe books is *Completely Perfect* by Felicity
Cloake, who also happens to be one of my favourite food writers.
She's the queen of executing the 'perfect' example of classic dishes,
and so often, when researching a recipe, I will read her 'perfect'
version to ensure I'm not playing too fast and loose with tradition.
Of course, I do tweak things, because I'm trying to hit certain
health targets. In the case of this lamb tagine, I've added chickpeas
for some complex carbs and fibre, but the main event here is zinc:
lots and lots of lovely zinc. Serve with some bulgur wheat, or rather
less conventionally, over a jacket potato.

Prep: 10 mins   Cooking: 2¼ hours   Serves: 4

2 tablespoons light olive oil
1 red onion, finely sliced
600g lean cubed lamb
½ teaspoon freshly ground black pepper
1 teaspoon ground cumin
1 teaspoon ground ginger
2 teaspoons paprika
½ teaspoon cayenne pepper
1 cinnamon stick
2 tablespoons tomato purée
25g fresh coriander, roughly chopped
salt
400g tin chickpeas, drained and rinsed
75g dried apricots, halved

Heat the oil in a large, heavy saucepan or casserole over a low
heat. Add the onion and sauté very gently for 5 minutes or so until
soft, then remove to a plate. Add the lamb and increase the heat

to medium–high. Fry off the lamb on all sides for 5 minutes or so, until golden brown. At this stage, drain off any excess oil. Now add the black pepper, cumin, ginger, paprika, cayenne pepper and the cinnamon stick and stir, then return the onions to the pan. Add the tomato purée, half the coriander and 400ml water, and stir thoroughly. Increase the heat to high until just about boiling, then reduce the heat to low. Cover loosely with a lid or foil and simmer for 1½ hours, stirring occasionally.

After this time, the meat should be getting nice and tender; taste and add salt as required. Remove the cinnamon stick, then add the chickpeas and apricots and simmer for a further 30 minutes. Add more water if it's looking too thick; you want a nice sauce remaining at the end.

Serve with the remaining coriander sprinkled over the top.

Nutrients (per serving)

Calories 487   *Protein* 34.3g (29%)

Total fat / saturated fat / omega-3 25.6g (47%) / 9.5g / 0.2g

Total carbs / sugar / fibre 30.8g (24%) / 14.3g / 6.8g

Vitamins and minerals A, B3, B12, phosphorus, selenium, zinc

LOWER-CALORIE MEALS

Raspberry Ripple Porridge

VE, GF (use GF-certified oats)

There's no more nutritious or filling way to kick off the day than with a bowl of porridge. I love this version because it has a thick, tart swirl of crushed raspberries through it, providing more fibre and polyphenols.

Prep: 5 mins   Cooking: 15 mins   Serves: 1

40g porridge oats
200ml semi-skimmed milk
1 teaspoon date syrup
½ teaspoon ground cinnamon

pinch of salt
50g fresh or defrosted frozen
   raspberries
1 tablespoon Greek yogurt

In a small saucepan over a medium heat, combine the oats, milk, date syrup, cinnamon and salt, and simmer gently for 10 minutes.

Meanwhile, place the raspberries in a bowl and mash up with a fork. If you have a microwave, you can cook them for 30 seconds and then mash, to make a kind of hot berry sauce. Pour the porridge into a bowl, swirl through the mashed raspberries and add the Greek yogurt on top to serve.

Nutrients (per serving)
Calories 311   *Protein* 15.5g (19%)
Total fat / saturated fat / omega-3 7.1g (20%) / 3.0g / 0.1g
Total carbs / sugar / fibre 48.1g (61%) / 16.8g / 8.2g
Vitamins and minerals B2, B12, D, calcium, phosphorus,
   manganese

Rainbow Vegetable Crustless Quiche

GF

If you love quiche but can't be bothered with the pastry, then this lower-calorie version is a good alternative. It's important to properly sauté all the vegetables first to ensure there's not too much liquid left, as that could make the quiche watery. This makes a tasty lunch, paired with a leafy green salad and a simple vinaigrette dressing (olive oil, apple cider vinegar, mixed dried herbs, Dijon mustard and salt and pepper).

Prep: 10 mins   Cooking: 50 mins   Serves: 4

4 large eggs
250ml milk
salt and freshly ground black pepper
75g frozen peas
1 tablespoon light olive oil
1 small red onion, finely sliced
½ red pepper, deseeded and finely sliced
75g broccoli, cut into tiny florets
100g tinned cannellini beans, drained and rinsed
50g Parmesan, grated

Preheat the oven to 180°C/gas mark 6 and line a deep 20cm × 15cm baking tin with baking parchment, making sure the parchment comes up higher than the top of the tin.

Whisk together the eggs and milk in a jug and season really well with salt and pepper.

Defrost the peas by covering with boiling water, then drain.

Now heat the oil in a large frying pan over a medium heat. Add the onion, red pepper and broccoli and slowly fry for about

5 minutes until soft. Add the peas and beans and cook gently for a further 5 minutes. Everything should be softened but not browned.

Now place the vegetables in the prepared tin, then pour over the egg and milk mixture. Top with the grated Parmesan and bake for 40 minutes until firm and nicely browned on top. Leave to cool slightly before lifting out of the tin. Cut into quarters and serve.

Nutrients (per serving)

Calories 247   *Protein* 15.0g (24%)

Total fat / saturated fat / omega-3 13.4g (48%) / 5.0g / 0.1g

Total carbs / sugar / fibre 17.2g (28%) / 6.1g / 3.3g

Vitamins and minerals A, B12, C, calcium, selenium, zinc

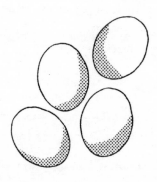

Borlotti Bean and Bacon Soup with Savoy Cabbage and Quinoa

DF, GF

This is a delicious and nourishing soup, and the thinking behind it was to introduce the idea of using bacon as a flavouring element. We know that we should minimise meat in our diets, especially processed meats like bacon, ham and chorizo, but that doesn't mean we have to eliminate them altogether. They are so tasty, and can be used in small amounts to flavour dishes, rather than being the main event. This soup also happens to be very nutritionally balanced, and still comes in under 400 calories.

Prep: 10 mins   Cooking: 25 mins   Serves: 2 (generously)

3 streaky bacon rashers (65g), sliced
250g savoy cabbage, finely sliced
400g tin borlotti beans, drained and rinsed
50g quinoa, rinsed thoroughly
750ml (1⅓ pints) vegetable stock, made from 1 cube
2 teaspoons apple cider vinegar
salt and freshly ground black pepper

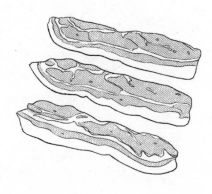

Heat a large saucepan over a medium heat and add the bacon. Fry for a few minutes until most of the fat has been released but the bacon is not browned. Add the cabbage and give it all a good stir. Now add the beans and the quinoa and pour over the stock. Add the apple cider vinegar and season very well with salt and pepper.

Bring to the boil, then reduce the heat to low and simmer for 20 minutes. Serve immediately. Any leftovers will keep nicely in the fridge for a couple of days.

Nutrients (per serving)

Calories 396   *Protein* 18.2g (16%)

Total fat / saturated fat / omega-3 15.7g (36%) / 0.3g / 0.1g

Total carbs / sugar / fibre 48.0g (48%) / 3.4g / 5.6g

Vitamins and minerals C, B6, B9, copper, potassium, zinc

Spinach, Squash and Red Onion Salad with Halloumi Croutons and a Sweet Chilli Dressing

GF

I don't know about you, but my mouth is watering just thinking about this salad. As this is a lower-calorie dish, the halloumi serves as crunchy croutons rather than being in huge slabs, but you'll still get all the squeaky saltiness. A quick tip on the butternut squash: this uses about half a small one, but roast the whole thing. You can keep the extra in the fridge to have in salads later in the week, or blend it into a vegetable soup.

Prep: 15 mins   Cooking: 40 mins plus cooling time   Serves: 2

300g butternut squash, deseeded and cut into 3cm cubes
1 small red onion, cut into chunks
1 tablespoon extra virgin olive oil
salt and freshly ground black pepper
100g halloumi, cut into 2cm cubes
130g baby spinach leaves

For the dressing
2 tablespoons Thai sweet chilli sauce
1 garlic clove, finely grated
2cm piece of fresh root ginger, peeled and finely grated
1 teaspoon fish sauce (omit, to make this VE)
juice of 1 lime

Preheat the oven to 200°C/gas mark 7.

Place the butternut squash cubes and red onion in a baking tray. Drizzle with the olive oil and season with salt and pepper, then roast for 30 minutes. Once cooked, remove from the oven and allow to cool to room temperature.

Make the dressing by combining all the ingredients in a small airtight container and giving it a good shake. Set aside.

Place a non-stick frying pan over a medium heat and add the halloumi cubes. Fry for a minute or so on each side, tossing them around in the pan to get as many sides golden as possible. Remove from the heat and set aside.

To assemble the salad, place the spinach leaves in a large salad bowl, then pour over the dressing and toss well to coat. Arrange the butternut squash and onions over the top, then sprinkle over the halloumi croutons. Eat immediately.

Nutrients (per serving)

Calories 365   *Protein* 15.2% (15%)

Total fat / saturated fat / omega-3 21.0g (52%) / 8.5g / 0.3g

Total carbs / sugar / fibre 33.1g (33%) / 9.6g / 6.6g

Vitamins and minerals B9, C, E, calcium, magnesium, manganese, phosphorus

---

Smoked Mackerel Pâté on Toast with Watercress and an Egg

—

If you follow me on Instagram, you'll know that smoked mackerel often crops up in my recipes. It's such an easy way to top up your omega-3 if you are feeling a bit lazy, as there's no need to cook it. I've been making this healthy smoked mackerel pâté for years, and this is often how I eat it – with toasted wholegrain sourdough toast, some kind of green leaf and a fried egg on top. This recipe makes a whole bowl of smoked mackerel pâté, but the nutritional breakdown here is based on having a 75g portion, so keep the rest in an airtight container in the fridge for future meals – breakfast, lunch or dinner!

Prep: 10 mins   Cooking: 0 mins   Serves: 1

1 egg
1 slice of good-quality wholegrain sourdough bread
handful of watercress
salt and freshly ground black pepper

For the smoked mackerel pâté (makes 3 portions)
300g pack of smoked mackerel fillets, skin removed and
    flesh flaked
3 tablespoons Greek yogurt
3 spring onions, finely sliced
juice of ½ lemon
freshly ground black pepper

To make the pâté, place all the ingredients in a bowl and thoroughly mash together with a fork.

Now take a good-quality non-stick frying pan (so no oil is needed) and fry the egg to your liking.

Toast the sourdough bread and spread with a portion of the smoked mackerel pâté. Top with the watercress and place the fried egg on top. Season with salt and pepper and serve. The rest of the pâté will keep in an airtight container for 2–3 days.

Nutrients (per serving)

Calories 387   *Protein* 29.2g (31%)

Total fat / saturated fat / omega-3 11.5g (27%) / 3.3g / 1.2g

Total carbs / sugar / fibre 41.0g (42%) / 4.3g / 2.1g

Vitamins and minerals B2, B12, D, potassium, selenium, zinc

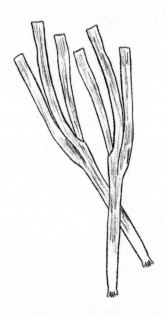

Spaghetti with Peas, Asparagus and Hot-smoked Salmon

—

Boy, oh boy – this may be a low-calorie recipe, but I'm telling you your taste buds are in for a treat! I could not be happier with this creation: complex carbs from the wholemeal spaghetti, protein and omega-3 from the oily fish, prebiotics from the asparagus, and a multitude of vitamins and minerals from the peas and lemon juice. A meal made in nutritional heaven.

Prep: 10 mins   Cooking: 15 mins   Serves: 2

100g wholemeal spaghetti
125g asparagus tips, sliced diagonally
100g frozen peas
50g cream cheese
juice of ½ lemon
salt and freshly ground black pepper
100g hot-smoked salmon, any skin removed and flesh flaked
35g Parmesan, grated
small handful of dill, chopped (optional)

Cook the spaghetti in a large saucepan of boiling water, according to the packet instructions.

Meanwhile, heat a smaller saucepan of water and, when boiling, add the asparagus and peas. Cook for 2–3 minutes, then drain, retaining a couple of tablespoons of water in the pan. Place the drained vegetables in a bowl of cold water; this will help them retain their colour and crunch.

Place the same saucepan over a low heat and add the cream cheese to the retained water. Bring to a simmer, then drain the vegetables once more and add to the pan. Stir in the lemon juice and season well with salt and pepper. Now add the flaked hot-smoked salmon and stir gently to combine.

When the spaghetti is ready, drain it, then return to the empty pan. Pour over the sauce and stir through. Divide between two serving bowls and sprinkle over the Parmesan and dill (if using).

Nutrients (per serving)

Calories 396   *Protein* 29.6g (30%)

Total fat / saturated fat / omega-3 10.9g (24%) / 4.7g / 0.9g

Total carbs / sugar / fibre 48.0g (46%) / 2.8g / 6.9g

Vitamins and minerals B12, C, D, iron, magnesium, selenium, zinc

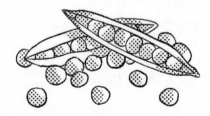

Roast Chicken with Herby Harissa Puy Lentils

DF, GF

Roast chicken is a midweek box-ticker – minimum effort, maximum flavour and everyone loves it. This version is a one-dish wonder, as the herby, spicy Puy lentils bubble away underneath while the bird roasts. If you are trying to keep the calories down, remove the skin from your portion. Serve with a nice big bowl of steamed green veg (savoy cabbage goes particularly well) for a complete meal under 500 calories.

Prep: 10 mins   Cooking: 1hr 40 mins   Serves: 4

- 1 medium chicken (1.5kg)
- 1 teaspoon light olive oil
- salt and freshly ground black pepper
- 1 tablespoon neutral oil
- 1 large onion, sliced
- 3 garlic cloves, roughly chopped
- 200g dried Puy lentils, rinsed
- 2 tablespoons harissa paste
- 15g flat-leaf parsley, chopped
- 10g mint leaves, chopped
- 600ml chicken stock, made from 1 cube
- 1 lemon, halved

Preheat the oven to 180°C/gas mark 6.

Rub the chicken all over with the olive oil and season the skin well with salt and pepper.

Heat the neutral oil in an ovenproof casserole dish over a low heat. Add the onion and sauté gently for 10 minutes until nicely softened.

Add the garlic and sauté for a further 2–3 minutes, then add the lentils. Stir well, then add the harissa paste, herbs and stock. Stir everything thoroughly to combine and season really well with salt and pepper. Place the lemon halves at either end of the casserole, then position the seasoned chicken in the middle and put in the oven to roast for 1 hour 20 minutes.

After this time, take the chicken out and check it's cooked by piercing the thigh with a sharp knife to ensure the juices are running clear. If not, return the chicken to the oven for a further 10–15 minutes. When it's cooked, remove from the oven and lift the chicken out of the casserole, tipping any juices from the cavity into the lentils. Place the chicken on a carving board to rest.

Remove the lemon halves from the casserole and give the lentils a stir. Taste for seasoning and add more salt or pepper if needed. Divide the lentils between four large bowls, then carve the chicken and place on top to serve.

Nutrients (per serving)

Calories 442 (skin removed)   *Protein* 48.5g (44%)

Total fat / saturated fat / omega-3 10.2g (21%) / 1.7g / 0.5g

Total carbs / sugar / fibre 38.9g (35%) / 3.5g / 6.5g

Vitamins and minerals A, B vitamins, K, this contain lots of minerals, in particular selenium and zinc

---

Hake Pomodoro with White Beans

DF, GF

The inspiration for this recipe was the flavours of bruschetta: ripe tomatoes, a punch of garlic and fresh basil. The hake fillets soak up all the beautiful flavours, and with the addition of white beans (I used cannellini), it's transformed into a wonderful, balanced, nutritious low-calorie meal that delivers a whole host of vitamins and minerals, and omega-3 too.

Prep: 10 mins   Cooking: 20 mins   Serves: 2

400g tin of white beans, drained and rinsed
150g vine or cherry tomatoes, chopped
10g basil leaves, chopped
2 garlic cloves, finely grated
2 tablespoons extra virgin olive oil
salt and freshly ground black pepper
2 × 140g hake fillets

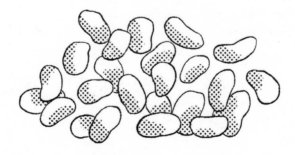

Preheat the oven to 200°C/gas mark 7.

In a bowl, combine the beans, tomatoes, basil, garlic, olive oil and a generous pinch of salt and pepper. Mix everything together with your fingers; you can squish the beans a bit to get the flavours really marrying. If you have time, leave the bowl to sit for half an hour or so, and the flavours will develop even more.

Now take a large piece of foil and spread the bean mixture over the foil. Place the hake fillets on top and season the top of the fillets with more salt and pepper. Fold the foil over and turn in the sides to make a sealed foil envelope. Place in the hot oven and bake for 20 minutes. Serve immediately with some crunchy green beans on the side.

Nutrients (per serving)

Calories 380   *Protein* 32.8g (34%)

Total fat / saturated fat / omega-3 14.7g (34%) / 21.0g / 0.4g

Total carbs / sugar / fibre 29.5g (32%) / 2.4g / 6.8g

Vitamins and minerals B12, E, K, this provides a good range
of minerals, including iodine, magnesium, manganese
and selenium

SMART SNACKS AND SWEET STUFF

Peanut Butter and Chia Seed Banana Bread

VE

Banana bread is not only foolproof, it's also one of the healthiest bakes out there, and this one is supercharged with goodness from wholemeal flour, peanut butter and chia seeds. I can't think of a better way to use up bananas that are a little past their best.

Prep: 10 mins   Cooking: 1 hour   Serves: 8

40g unsalted butter, softened, plus extra for greasing
150g wholemeal flour, plus extra for dusting
100g light brown sugar
1 large egg
100ml milk
2½ teaspoons baking powder
2 teaspoons ground cinnamon
2 ripe bananas, roughly mashed
2 tablespoons crunchy peanut butter
2 tablespoons chia seeds

Preheat the oven to 175°C/gas mark 5½ and grease and flour a 450g loaf tin.

Cream together the butter and sugar in a large bowl, then add the egg and milk and combine with a hand mixer. Sift in the flour (returning any wheatgerm to the bowl), followed by the baking powder and cinnamon. Stir to incorporate.

In a smaller bowl, combine the mashed bananas with the peanut butter. Add to the cake mixture, along with the chia seeds, and stir gently to combine. Pour the batter into the prepared loaf tin and bake for 1 hour.

When it's done it will be risen and golden on top. Allow to cool a little before turning out of the tin. It's lovely eaten warm but will keep for several days in an airtight container.

Nutrients (per serving)

Calories 227   *Protein* 4.8g (9%)

Total fat / saturated fat / omega-3 7.9g (32%) / 3.3g / 0.5g

Total carbs / sugar / fibre 36.1g (59%) / 16.2g / 2.7g

Vitamins and minerals B vitamins, magnesium, potassium, selenium

---

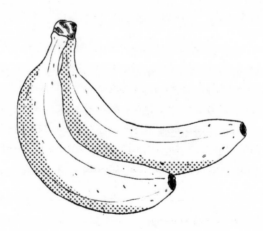

Healthy Mixed Berry Crumble

VG, VE, DF

This delicious, fruity, crumbly pud ticks all the boxes, as far as I'm concerned. My midlife palate prefers this served with a dollop of creamy Greek yogurt – not for your VG/DF folk, of course – but it goes equally well with ice cream or custard; those just add a few more calories! You can use honey or maple syrup instead of date syrup, if you prefer.

Prep: 10 mins   Cooking: 25 mins   Serves: 8

50g coconut oil
75g rolled oats
30g flaked almonds
30g sunflower seeds
70g wholemeal flour

1 teaspoon ground cinnamon
50g light brown sugar
3 tablespoons date syrup
500g frozen mixed berries

Preheat the oven to 180°C/gas mark 6.

To make the topping, melt the coconut oil in a small saucepan over a low heat. Remove from the heat and add the oats, almonds, sunflower seeds, flour, cinnamon, sugar and date syrup. Now place the frozen berries in a single layer in a shallow baking dish and cover with the oaty topping. Bake for 25 minutes until the fruit is sticky and bubbling and the topping has gone nice and crisp, then serve with your chosen accompaniments.

Nutrients (per serving)

Calories 240   *Protein* 4.6g (7%)

Total fat / saturated fat / omega-3 11.3g (40%) / 5.9g / 0.1g

Total carbs / sugar / fibre 33.1g (53%) / 16.2g / 4.6g

Vitamins and minerals B1, B2, E, copper, magnesium, manganese

---

Oaty Fruit Slices

VE

The mistake many people make when trying to be healthy is to cut out all 'treats' in the form of sugar and fat. The problem is that you are not going to stop wanting them – and really, why should you? There's no need to be so extreme. Health doesn't work that way; it responds better to consistency and moderation. This recipe does contain some butter and some sugar (in the form of my beloved date syrup), but there's also lots of fibre from the wholegrains and fruit, so you won't get that dreaded sugar spike. Enjoy!

Prep: 10 mins   Cooking: 45 mins   Serves: 12

100g pitted dates, chopped
75g dried apricots, chopped
75g soft dried figs, stalks removed, chopped
125g salted butter
50g date syrup (approx. 5 tablespoons)
200g rolled oats
50g mixed seeds
50g wholemeal flour
1 teaspoon ground cinnamon

Preheat the oven to 160°C/gas mark 4 and line a 25cm × 20cm baking tray with a strip of baking parchment.

Place the dried fruit in a small saucepan and cover with cold water. Bring to the boil, then turn the heat down to low and simmer for 20 minutes until soft. Remove from the heat and allow to cool slightly, then mash with a fork.

Place the butter and date syrup in a separate small saucepan and melt gently over a low heat, mixing well.

The Recipes

Combine all the dry ingredients in a large bowl. Pour in the butter and syrup mixture and mix well, then add the mashed fruits and stir through. Spread out in the prepared baking tray and press down gently, then bake for 25 minutes.

Allow to cool completely, then cut into 12 equal pieces.

Nutrients (per serving)

Calories 4.9g (7%)   *Protein* 4.9g (7%)

Total fat / saturated fat / omega-3 11.9g (43%) / 5.7g / 0.1g

Total carbs / sugar / fibre 31.7g (50%) / 14.1g / 4.4g

Vitamins and minerals A, B1, E, magnesium, manganese,
 phosphorus

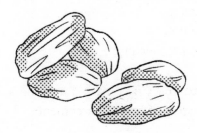

Prune Power Balls

VG, VE, DF, GF

I know prunes can be a bit of a turn-off – all that chat about keeping you regular! – but if you just think of them as dried plums, they are a bit more tempting. The truth is, they are really good for you, with antioxidants, fibre, and a whole range of vitamins and minerals, as well as being a good plant-based source of iodine. These are best kept in the fridge and eaten with a cup of tea for a healthy, fibre-rich snack.

Prep: 15 mins   Cooking: 0 mins   Portions: makes 12 balls

200g soft, pitted prunes
75g walnuts
4 tablespoons ground almonds, plus more to coat
juice of 1 lime
1 tablespoon maple syrup
1 teaspoon ground ginger
1 teaspoon ground cinnamon
a pinch of salt

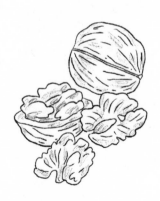

The Recipes

Place all the ingredients in a food processor and blend on high until well combined. The consistency should be quite stiff, as you need to roll it into balls. If it's too stiff to blend properly, add a drop of water; if it's too wet, add more ground almonds.

Place some more ground almonds in a small bowl, then take a dessertspoon-sized amount of the prune mixture and drop it into the ground almonds. Move around gently to coat, then pick it up and lightly roll into a ball.

Repeat until you have approximately 12 balls. Keep in an airtight container in the fridge for up to a week.

Nutrients (per serving)

Calories 99   *Protein* 2.1g (8%)

Total fat / saturated fat / omega-3 6.2g (52%) / 0.6g / 0.6g

Total carbs / sugar / fibre 10.9g (40%) / 5.9g / 1.9g

Vitamins and minerals B2, E, K, copper, iodine, magnesium, manganese

---

Nut Butter-stuffed Frozen Dates

VG, VE, DF, GF

This is my favourite snack. Honestly, if you need a sweet fix, this is the healthiest way to do it, and because you eat them from frozen, you can make a big batch, stick them in the freezer, and they are there to do service whenever the munchies hit.

Prep: 10 mins   Cooking: 0 mins   Portions: 12 x 1 date

- 12 Medjool dates
- 12 teaspoons good-quality peanut butter (or make the Omega-3 Nut Butter on page 151)

Open up the first date and remove the pit. Fill the cavity with 1 teaspoon of nut butter. Pinch the sides back together and place in an airtight container. Repeat until all the dates are filled, then place the container in the freezer.

These are best eaten straight from frozen.

Nutrients (per serving)

Calories 98   *Protein* 1.7g (6%)

Total fat / saturated fat / omega-3 2.7g (23%) / 0.4g / 0.0g

Total carbs / sugar / fibre 19.2g (71%) / 16.4g / 2.0g

Vitamins and minerals B3, B5, B6, copper, magnesium, manganese

---

Hot-smoked Salmon Smash-up

GF

I'm a massive fan of smoked mackerel pâté, and this hot-smoked salmon version, introduced to me by my friend and fellow food writer Ghillie James, is perhaps even better. It's simplicity itself, and an absolute powerhouse of omega-3 and protein. Serve on nice crusty brown toast, or on little crackers or blinis as a healthy canapé.

Prep: 5 mins   Cooking: 0 mins   Serves: 2

150g hot-smoked salmon, any skin removed
2 tablespoons Greek yogurt
2 spring onions, finely sliced
1 tablespoon dill, chopped (optional)
squeeze of lemon juice
freshly ground black pepper

Place the salmon in a bowl and mash up with a fork. Add the rest of the ingredients and mix well to combine. Store in an airtight container in the fridge. This will keep for three days.

Nutrients (per serving)

Calories 132   *Protein* 20.2g (64%)

Total fat / saturated fat / omega-3 4.4g (30%) / 1.0g / 0.5g

Total carbs / sugar / fibre 2.1g (6%) / 0.9g / 0.5g

Vitamins and minerals B12, D, K, calcium, phosphorus,
   selenium

Cheesy Chive Wholemeal Scones

VE

My love of a cheese scone knows no bounds, and so I definitely had a vested interest in coming up with a healthier version! The tweaks I've made here are subbing in some wholemeal flour for the usual white flour and using olive oil instead of butter. They are very moreish, so my tip is to eat one fresh from the oven and freeze the rest. If you cut them in half before freezing, you can just pop them in the toaster when you fancy a savoury snack.

Prep: 15 mins   Cooking: 15 mins   Portions: makes 12 scones

200g self-raising flour
150g wholemeal flour
2 teaspoons baking powder
1 teaspoon salt
handful of chives (10g), chopped
60ml extra virgin olive oil
2 eggs
75ml milk
3 teaspoons Dijon mustard
60g mature Cheddar, grated

Preheat the oven to 220°C/gas mark 9.

Sift the flours and baking powder into a large mixing bowl, adding any bran left in the sieve back into the bowl. Stir in the salt and chopped chives.

In another bowl, whisk together the olive oil, eggs and milk with a fork. Now gradually add this mixture to the dry ingredients, mixing well until it comes together as a dough.

Divide the mixture into 12 equal-sized balls of approx. 50g each, and place in a 12-hole muffin tin. Spread some Dijon mustard on the top of each one and then top with the grated cheese. Bake for 15 minutes.

Delicious eaten warm, or allow to cool on a wire rack and either freeze or keep in an airtight container for 2–3 days.

Nutrients (per serving)

Calories 181   *Protein* 5.7g (13%)

Total fat / saturated fat / omega-3 8.0g (39%) / 2.0g / 0.1g

Total carbs / sugar / fibre 21.9g (48%) / 0.5g / 1.9g

Vitamins and minerals B1, B2, B9, calcium, phosphorus, selenium

---

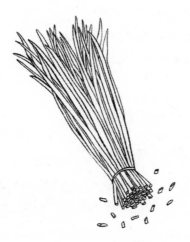

Super Seedy Crackers

VG, VE, DF

I must admit, I'm not usually one for making my own crackers. They fall into the same category as decent bread – so much easier to just buy! But on my Leith's course, we made a version of these seedy crackers, and they were so good that from time to time, I do make the effort! These are great with soup as an alternative to bread, and they provide fibre and plenty of plant-based omega-3.

Prep: 10 mins   Cooking: 40 mins   Portions: 30 × 15g crackers

- 65g sunflower seeds
- 45g flaxseeds
- 25g pumpkin seeds
- 20g sesame seeds
- 75g rolled oats
- 1 tablespoon chia seeds
- 2 tablespoons psyllium husk or wheatgerm
- 1 tablespoon dried mixed herbs
- ¾ teaspoon fine sea salt
- ½ teaspoon maple syrup
- 1½ tablespoons melted coconut oil

In a large bowl, combine all the dry ingredients.

In a small bowl, whisk together the maple syrup, coconut oil and 175ml water until fully combined. Add this mixture to the dry ingredients and mix until everything is completely combined and the dough becomes thick. If it is too stiff to roll, add another teaspoon of water.

Divide the dough in half and roll out each half between 2 pieces of baking parchment until very thin, about 2mm. Remove the top piece of parchment and leave uncovered on two baking sheets for a couple of hours to dry out a little.

Preheat the oven to 180°C/gas mark 6.

Place the crackers in the oven and bake for 25 minutes. Remove from the oven, and carefully turn over, peeling off the remaining baking parchment. Bake on the other side for a further 15 minutes until crisp. Allow the crackers to cool completely, then break into pieces and store in an airtight container for up to 3 weeks.

Nutrients (per serving)
Calories 48   *Protein* 1.7g (12%)
Total fat / saturated fat / omega-3 3.6g (62%) / 0.9g / 0.4g
Total carbs / sugar / fibre 3.1g (26%) / 0.2g / 1.3g
Vitamins and minerals B1, B6, E, magnesium, manganese, zinc

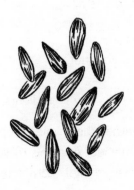

HEALTHY DRINKS

Zingy 'Get Going' Morning Tea

VE, DF, GF

If you aren't a coffee fan but still want something invigorating to get you up and running in the morning, then this is a fresh and fragrant alternative. The honey is optional if you want to keep sugar off the morning menu.

Prep: 5 mins   Cooking: 0 mins   Serves: 1

juice of ½ lemon
small handful of mint leaves
boiling water
1 teaspoon honey

Place the lemon juice in a mug. Gently crush the mint leaves in your hand, then add those to the mug as well. Pour over boiling water and add the honey, if using. Stir well and allow to steep for 5 minutes before drinking.

Nutrients (per serving)
Calories 30   *Protein* 0.3g (3%)
Total fat / saturated fat / omega-3 0.1g (3%) / 0.0g / 0.0g
Total carbs / sugar / fibre 8.3g (94%) / 6.4g / 0.5g
Vitamins and minerals C

Probiotic ACV Lemonade

VG, VE, DF, GF

This is grown-up lemonade that's good for the gut and super refreshing. You can adjust the maple syrup to taste; I don't like it sweet, but you might wish to add a little more.

Prep: 5 mins   Cooking: 0 mins   Serves: 1

juice of 1 lemon
1 tablespoon apple cider vinegar
1 teaspoon maple syrup
300ml sparkling water
ice, to serve

Place the lemon juice, apple cider vinegar and maple syrup in a tall glass and give it a good stir. Top up with the carbonated water and add a few ice cubes to serve.

Nutrients (per serving)
Calories 31   *Protein* 0.2g (2%)
Total fat / saturated fat / omega-3 0.1g (4%) / 0.0g / 0.0g
Total carbs / sugar / fibre 7.9g (94%) / 5.3g / 0.1g
Vitamins and minerals B2, C, calcium, magnesium, manganese

Ginger and Cinnamon Tea for Digestion

VG, VE, DF, GF

Ginger and cinnamon are both well known for their digestive properties, and they are put to good use here in a simple tea. An excellent early-evening option.

Prep: 5 mins   Cooking: 0 mins   Serves: 1

5cm piece of fresh root ginger, peeled and finely sliced
boiling water
1 cinnamon stick

Place the ginger in a mug and top up with boiling water. Use the cinnamon stick to muddle the ginger in the water. Let it sit for a few minutes, then drink.

Nutrients (per serving)

Calories 7   Protein 0.1g (5%)

Total fat / saturated fat / omega-3 0.1g (7%) / 0.0g / 0.0g

Total carbs / sugar / fibre 1.9g (88%) / 0.1g / 0.7g

Vitamins and minerals Manganese

Hibiscus Iced Tea for High Blood Pressure

VE, DF, GF

I'm not usually one for faffing around sourcing unusual ingredients, but if you suffer from high blood pressure or raised cholesterol, then it might be worth taking a few minutes online to buy some dried hibiscus flowers, as this iced tea can help with both issues.

Prep: 5 mins   Cooking: 0 mins   Serves: 2

1 tablespoon dried hibiscus flowers
1 star anise
2 teaspoons honey
squeeze of lime juice
ice cubes, to serve

Place all the ingredients in a jug with 500ml cold water. Mix well, then leave to chill in the fridge for at least an hour. Serve over ice.

Nutrients (per serving)

Calories 31   *Protein* 0.2g (3%)

Total fat / saturated fat / omega-3 0.1g (4%) / 0.0g / 0.0g

Total carbs / sugar / fibre 8.5g (93%) / 6.6g / 0.2g

Vitamins and minerals B1, C

Alcohol-free White Sangria

VG, VE, DF, GF

Having a party, but don't want a hangover afterwards? Make this. It's very low-calorie and full of fruity goodness. You can buy alcohol-free sparkling wines in most supermarkets now; there are a few different ones, including Nozeco, Noughty and Fizzero. You need the wine really cold to start with, as adding ice makes the fizz disappear.

Prep: 10 mins   Cooking: 0 mins   Serves: 12

150ml elderflower cordial
2 bottles of very cold alcohol-free sparkling wine
50g fresh root ginger, peeled and finely sliced
4 limes, thinly sliced into rounds
3 peaches, stoned and sliced
100g raspberries

Place the elderflower cordial in a large jug or punch bowl. Add the alcohol-free wine and gently stir. Add the ginger slices and fruit and serve immediately.

Nutrients (per serving)

Calories 65   *Protein* 0.5g (3%)

Total fat / saturated fat / omega-3 0.2g (3%) / 0.0g / 0.0g

Total carbs / sugar / fibre 15.4g (94%) / 12.6g / 1.2g

Vitamins and minerals C

Hydrating Watermelon Mocktail

VE, DF, GF

How much this makes does, obviously, depend on how big your watermelon is, and how much you choose to dilute it with sparkling water, but it's a really nice summery way to kick off a barbecue without the booze.

Prep: 10 mins   Cooking: 0 mins   Serves: about 10

1 small watermelon (2kg), skin and pips removed
1 tablespoon honey
juice of 2 limes
ice cubes
sparkling water, to top up

Cut the watermelon flesh into chunks and place in a blender. Pulse until smooth; you may have to do this in a few batches. Pass the resulting juice through a sieve and into a large jug. Add the honey and lime juice, and stir well. Pour into tall glasses, filling them halfway. Add a few ice cubes to each glass and top up with sparkling water, then serve.

Nutrients (per serving)

Calories 69   *Protein* 1.3g (6%)

Total fat / saturated fat / omega-3 0.3g (4%) / 0.0g / 0.0g

Total carbs / sugar / fibre 17.6g (90%) / 14.3g / 0.8g

Vitamins and minerals A, C, magnesium

Anti-inflammatory Evening Milk

VE, GF

If you like something warming and comforting in the evening, then try this to benefit from the fabulous anti-inflammatory properties of turmeric. Don't be put off by the black pepper; it just adds a low heat and is required to make the curcumin (the good stuff) in the turmeric bioavailable, which means it can be absorbed and used by the body.

Prep: 2 mins   Cooking: 3 mins   Serves: 1

250ml semi-skimmed milk (or non-dairy milk)
½ teaspoon ground turmeric
¼ teaspoon ground ginger
¼ teaspoon ground cinnamon
1 teaspoon honey
tiny pinch of freshly ground black pepper

Place all the ingredients in a small saucepan and whisk together. Heat until almost boiling, then serve.

Nutrients (per serving)

Calories 155   *Protein* 8.5g (24%)

Total fat / saturated fat / omega-3 5.0g (28%) / 3.1g / 0.0g

Total carbs / sugar / fibre 19.8g (48%) / 18.6g / 0.8g

Vitamins and minerals B12, D, calcium

Sleeping Potion

VG, VE, DF, GF

This night-time drink has all the sleep-inducing properties of chamomile tea, as well as the sleep-promoting compounds tryptophan, melatonin and magnesium, all found in almond milk. A natural way to get your body ready for bed.

Prep: 5 mins   Cooking: 0 mins   Serves: 1

100ml boiling water
1 chamomile teabag
300ml almond milk
½ teaspoon vanilla extract
1 teaspoon maple syrup

Heat the water in a small saucepan and, when boiling, add the tea bag. Reduce the heat to low and allow to steep for a minute, then remove the teabag. Add the remaining ingredients to the pan and mix well. Heat through and serve.

Nutrients (per serving)

Calories 176   *Protein* 9.9g (25%)

Total fat / saturated fat / omega-3 6.0g (31%) / 3.8g / 0.0g

Total carbs / sugar / fibre 19.6g (44%) / 19.4g / 0.0g

Vitamins and minerals D, E, calcium, magnesium

APPENDIX

A: NHS portion-size guide for fruit and vegetables

(Source: www.nhs.uk/live-well/eat-well/5-a-day/portion-sizes)

Everyone should have at least five portions of a variety of fruit and vegetables every day. An adult portion of fruit or vegetables is 80g. The guide below will give you an indication of the typical portion sizes for adults. Children should also eat at least five portions of a variety of fruit and vegetables a day. The amount of food a child needs varies with age, body size and levels of physical activity. As a rough guide, one portion is the amount they can fit in the palm of their hand.

Five-a-day fruit portions

Small-sized fresh fruit – A portion is two or more small fruits – for example, two plums, two satsumas, two kiwi fruits, three apricots, six lychees, seven strawberries or fourteen cherries.

Medium-sized fresh fruit – A portion is one piece of fruit, such as one apple, banana, pear, orange or nectarine.

Large fresh fruit – A portion is half a grapefruit, one slice of papaya, one slice of melon (5cm slice), one large slice of pineapple or two slices of mango (5cm slices).

Dried fruit – A portion of dried fruit is around 30g. This is about 1 heaped tablespoon of raisins, currants or sultanas, 1 tablespoon of mixed fruit, two figs, three prunes or a handful of dried banana chips. Note: Dried fruit can be high in sugar and can be bad for your teeth. Try to swap dried fruit for fresh fruit, especially between meals.

Tinned or canned fruit – A portion is roughly the same quantity of fruit that you would eat for a fresh portion, such as two pear or peach halves, six apricot halves or eight segments of tinned grapefruit. Choose fruit canned in natural juice rather than syrup.

Five-a-day vegetable portions

Green vegetables – A portion is two broccoli spears or 4 heaped tablespoons of cooked kale, spinach, spring greens or green beans.

Cooked vegetables – A portion is 3 heaped tablespoons of cooked vegetables, such as carrots, peas or sweetcorn, or eight cauliflower florets.

Salad vegetables – A portion is 1½ full-length celery sticks, a 5cm piece of cucumber, one medium tomato or seven cherry tomatoes.

Tinned and frozen vegetables – Roughly the same quantity as you would eat for a fresh portion. For example, 3 heaped tablespoons of tinned or frozen carrots, peas or sweetcorn count as one portion each. For tinned, choose those canned in water, with no added salt or sugar.

Pulses and beans – A portion is 3 heaped tablespoons of baked beans, haricot beans, kidney beans, cannellini beans, butter beans or chickpeas. Remember, however much you eat, beans and pulses count as a maximum of one of your five-a-day.

Potatoes – Potatoes don't count towards your five-a-day. This is the same for yams, cassava and plantain. They're classified nutritionally as a starchy food, because when eaten as part of a meal, they're usually used in place of other sources of starch, such as bread, rice or pasta. Although they don't count towards your five-a-day, potatoes do play an important role in your diet as a starchy food.

Five-a-day in juices and smoothies

Your combined total of drinks from fruit juice, vegetable juice and smoothies shouldn't be more than 150ml a day, which is a small glass.

Unsweetened 100% fruit juice, vegetable juice and smoothies can only ever count as a maximum of one portion of your five-a-day. For example, if you have two glasses of fruit juice and a smoothie in one day, that still only counts as one of your five-a-day. If you have 150ml of orange juice and a 150ml smoothie in one day, you'll have exceeded the recommendation by 150ml.

B: Aggregate Nutrient Density Index (ANDI) Sample Nutrient/Calorie-density Scores

(Source: www.drfuhrman.com/blog/128/andi-food-scores-rating-the-nutrient-density-of-foods)

Kale	1000	Courgettes	164
Spring greens	1000	Artichokes	145
Watercress	1000	Blueberries	132
Swiss chard	895	Iceberg lettuce	127
Pak choy	865	Grapes	119
Spinach	707	Pomegranates	119
Rocket	604	Cantaloupe	118
Romaine	510	Onions	109
Brussels sprouts	490	Flaxseeds	103
Carrots	458	Oranges	98
Cabbage	434	Edamame	98
Broccoli	340	Cucumbers	87
Cauliflower	315	Tofu	82
Bell peppers	265	Sesame Seeds	74
Asparagus	205	Lentils	72
Mushrooms	238	Peaches	65
Tomatoes	186	Sunflower seeds	64
Strawberries	182	Kidney beans	64
Sweet potatoes	181	Green peas	63

Appendix

Cherries	55	Brown rice	28
Pineapple	54	White Potatoes	28
Apples	53	Low-fat plain yogurt	28
Mangoes	53	Cashews	27
Peanut butter	51	Chicken breast	24
Corn	45	Minced beef, 85% lean	21
Pistachio nuts	37	Feta	20
Oatmeal	36	French fries	12
Prawns	36	White pasta	11
Salmon	34	Cheddar cheese	11
Eggs	31	Apple juice	11
Milk (semi-skimmed)	31	Olive oil	10
Walnuts	30	White bread	9
Bananas	30	Vanilla ice cream	9
Wholegrain bread	30	Corn tortilla chips	7
Almonds	28	Cola	1
Avocados	28		

Conversion Charts

Weight

10g	¼oz	225g	8oz
15g	½oz	250g	9oz
25/30g	1oz	300g	10½oz
40g	1½oz	350g	12oz
50g	1¾oz	375g	13oz
55g	2oz	400g	14oz
70g	2½oz	450g	1lb
85g	3oz	500g	1lb 2oz
100g	3½oz	600g	1lb 5oz
115g	4oz	750g	1lb 10oz
150g	5½oz	900g	2lb
200g	7oz	1kg	2lb 4oz

Volume: liquids

5ml	–	1 tsp
15ml	½fl oz	1 tbsp
30ml	1fl oz	2 tbsp
60ml	2fl oz	¼ cup
75ml	2½fl oz	⅓ cup
120ml	4fl oz	½ cup
150ml	5fl oz	⅔ cup
175ml	6fl oz	¾ cup
250ml	8fl oz	1 cup
350ml	12fl oz	1½ cups
500ml	18fl oz	2 cups
1 litre	1¾ pints	4 cups

Appendix

Volume: dry ingredients – an approximate guide

Flour	125g	1 cup
Butter	225g	1 cup (2 sticks)
Breadcrumbs (dried)	125g	1 cup
Nuts	125g	1 cup
Seeds	160g	1 cup
Dried fruit	150g	1 cup
Dried pulses (large)	175g	1 cup
Grains & small pulses	200g	1 cup

Oven temperatures

°C	with fan	°F	gas mark
110°C	90°C	225°F	¼
120°C	100°C	250°F	½
140°C	120°C	275°F	1
150°C	130°C	300°F	2
160°C	140°C	325°F	3
180°C	160°C	350°F	4
190°C	170°C	375°F	5
200°C	180°C	400°F	6
220°C	200°C	425°F	7
230°C	210°C	450°F	8
240°C	220°C	475°F	9

Length

1cm	½ inch		8cm	3¼ inches
2.5cm	1 inch		10cm	4 inches
3cm	1¼ inches		20cm	8 inches
5cm	2 inches		25cm	10 inches

Acknowledgements

Writing a book is not just a personal endeavour, it's something all my family and friends undertake with me. Whether as sounding boards, recipe-testers, guinea pigs or unpaid editors, many of my nearest and dearest have been part of the process of creating this book – even if it's just tearing me away from my desk for an hour or two.

I'd like to make a few special mentions, however, to those that went beyond the call of duty with very little by way of reward. Specifically my fabulous recipe-testers, who do it all for free, and without whose input the recipes wouldn't be half as good. Marie, Anjli, Hilary, Katie, Sara, Louise, Joanne, Emma and Vikki: you rock!

Another big thank you has to go to my mum, Stephanie, my most trusted (unpaid) editor. With a command of English second to none and a hawk's eye for detail, my copy is all the cleaner once it has been passed by you.

I wish to thank my brilliant agent Antony Topping at Greene & Heaton, without whom I wouldn't be writing books at all, and my excellent team at Headline Home, led by the wonderful Lindsey Evans, who has such confidence in my ability to pull a decent book out of the bag. You are fabulous humans. Thanks for bringing my words to life.

And finally, a shout-out to my ever-supportive friends and family: the 'Gorgeous Babes' Lisa, Jodi, Vics, Jane and Antonia for your endless drum-banging on my behalf; my fellow food writer Ghillie James, who is a constant source of ideas and inspiration; and last but not least, my husband Rich and kids Rufus and Roxana, for being at the sharp end of my recipe-testing, good and bad!

References

1 Kopp, W. *et al*. 'How Western diet and lifestyle drive the pandemic of obesity and civilization diseases'. *Diabetes, Metabolic Syndrome and Obesity: Targets And Therapy*, vol. 12, 24 October 2019, pp. 2221–36.

2 Public Health England. 'PHE publishes latest data on nation's diet'. 16 March 2018. www.gov.uk

3 Public Health England. 'Scale of the obesity problem'. 31 March 2017. www.gov.uk

4 Fadnes, L. T. *et al*. 'Estimating impact of food choices on life expectancy: A modelling study'. *PLOS Medicine*, vol. 19, no. 3, 8 February 2022.

5 Public Health England. *Government Dietary Recommendations*. August 2016.

6 Spector, T. D. *Spoon-Fed: Why almost everything we've been told about food is wrong*. Vintage, 2016.

7 Hayhoe, R. *et al*. 'Cross-sectional associations of schoolchildren's fruit and vegetable consumption, and meal choices, with their mental well-being: A cross-sectional study'. *BMJ Nutrition, Prevention & Health*, September 2021.

8 Derbyshire, E. 'Micronutrient intakes of British adults across mid-life: A secondary analysis of the UK national diet and nutrition survey'. *Frontiers in Nutrition*, vol. 5, 2018.

9 'Middle age may be much more stressful now than in the '90s'. sciencedaily.com, 7 May 2020.

10 Nowson, C. *et al*. 'Protein requirements and recommendations for older people: A Review'. *Nutrients*, vol. 7, no. 8, 14 August 2015.

11 Morris, S. *et al*. 'Inadequacy of protein intake in older UK adults'. *Geriatrics*, vol. 5, no. 1, 12 February 2020.

12 Russell, R. M. 'Factors in aging that effect the bioavailability of nutrients'. *The Journal of Nutrition*, vol. 131, no. 4, April 2001.

13 Bullamore, R. J. *et al*. 'Effect of Age on Calcium Absorption'. *The Lancet*, vol. 297, no. 7672, September 1970, pp. 535–7.

14 Rosie Greenaway. 'Pandemic prompts 19% rise in supplement consumption'. naturalproductsonline.co.uk, 8 February 2021.

15 Grand View Research. *Dietary Supplements Market Size, Share, Trends and Analysis Report, 2022–2030*. grandviewresearch.com

16 Community Research. *Food Supplements Consumer Research: Final Report for Food Standards Agency*. food.gov.uk, May 2018.

17 Zhang, F. F. *et al*. 'Health effects of vitamin and mineral supplements'. *BMJ*, vol. 369, June 2020.

References

18 Nierenberg, C. 'Getting too much of vitamins and minerals'. webmd.com, 6 March 2022.

19 Miller, P.E. *et al.* 'Low-calorie sweeteners and body weight and composition: A meta-analysis of randomized controlled trials and prospective cohort studies'. *American journal of Clinical Nutrition*, vol. 100, no. 3, September 2014, pp. 765–77.

20 Yang, Q. 'Artificial Sweeteners and the Neurobiology of Sugar Cravings'. *Yale Journal of Biology and Medicine*, vol. 83, no. 2, June 2010, pp. 101–8.

21 Suez, J. *et al.* 'Artificial sweeteners induce glucose intolerance by altering the gut microbiota'. *Nature*, vol. 514, no. 7521, 9 October 2014, pp. 181–6.

22 Ray, J. *et al.* 'Effects of stevia rebaudiana on glucose homeostasis, blood pressure and inflammation: A critical review of past and current research evidence'. *International Journal of Clinical Research & Trials*, vol. 5, 22 January 2020.

23 Ajami, M. *et al.* 'Effects of stevia on glycemic and lipid profile of type 2 diabetic patients: A randomized controlled trial'. *Avicenna Journal of Phytomedicine*, vol. 10, no. 2, March–April 2020, pp. 118–27.

24 Becker S. L. *et al.* 'Effect of stevia on the gut microbiota and glucose tolerance in a murine model of diet-induced obesity'. *FEMS Microbiology Ecology*, vol. 96, no. 6, 1 June 2020.

25 Arnett, D. K. *et al.* 'ACC/AHA guideline on the primary prevention of cardiovascular disease: A report of the American College of Cardiology/American Heart Association Task Force on Clinical Practice Guidelines'. *Circulation*, vol. 140, no. 11, 17 March 2019.

26 Bhanpuri, N. H. *et al.* 'Cardiovascular disease risk factor responses to a type 2 diabetes care model including nutritional ketosis induced by sustained carbohydrate restriction at 1 Year: An open label, non-randomized, controlled study - cardiovascular diabetology'. *Cardiovascular Diabetology*, vol. 17, no. 56, 1 May 2018.

27 British Nutrition Foundation. 'Protein'. nutrition.org.uk.

28 Papier, K. *et al.* 'Meat consumption and risk of 25 common conditions: Outcome-wide analyses in 475,000 men and women in the UK Biobank Study'. *BMC Medicine*, vol. 19, no. 53, 2 March 2021.

29 NHS. 'Meat in your diet'. nhs.uk

30 Harvard Health Publishing. 'Eat more plant-based proteins to boost longevity'. health.harvard.edu, 1 November 2020.

31 Sun, Q. *et al.* 'A prospective study of trans fatty acids in erythrocytes and risk of coronary heart disease'. *Circulation*, vol. 115, no. 14, 10 April 2007, pp. 1858–65.

32 Heileson J. L. 'Dietary saturated fat and heart disease: A narrative review'. *Nutrition Reviews*, vol. 78, no. 6, 1 June 2020, pp. 474–85.

33 Ebbeling, C. *et al.* 'Effects of a low-carbohydrate diet on insulin-resistant dyslipoproteinemia—a randomized controlled feeding trial'. *American Journal of Clinical Nutrition*, vol. 115, no. 1, 1 January 2022, pp. 154–62.

34 British Dietetic Association (BDA). 'Omega-3 Food Fact Sheet'. bda.uk.com, 2021.

References

35 Russo, G. L. 'Dietary N-6 and N-3 polyunsaturated fatty acids'. *Biochemical Pharmacology*, vol. 77, no. 6, November 2008, pp. 937–46.

36 British Nutrition Foundation. 'Fat'. nutrition.org.uk.

37 Drouin-Chartier, J. P. *et al.* 'Egg consumption and risk of cardiovascular disease: Three large prospective US cohort studies, systematic review, and updated meta-analysis'. *BMJ*, vol. 368, 4 March 2020.

38 Schmidt K. A. *et al.* 'Impact of low-fat and full-fat dairy foods on fasting lipid profile and blood pressure: Exploratory endpoints of a randomized controlled trial'. *American Journal of Clinical Nutrition*, vol. 114, no. 3, 1 September 2021, 882–92.

39 Wang, L. *et al.* 'A moderate-fat diet with one avocado per day increases plasma antioxidants and decreases the oxidation of small, dense LDL in adults with overweight and obesity: A randomized controlled trial'. *Journal of Nutrition*, vol. 150, no. 2, 1 February 2020, pp. 276–84.

40 Jackson C. *et al.* 'Long-term associations of nut consumption with body weight and obesity'. *American Journal of Clinical Nutrition*, vol. 100, July 2014.

41 Reynolds, A. N. *et al.* 'Dietary fibre and wholegrains in diabetes management: Systematic review and Meta-analyses'. *PLOS Medicine*, 6 March 2020.

42 The Food & Drink Federation. 'Action on fibre'. fdf.org.uk.

43 Jacka, F. N. *et al.* 'A randomised controlled trial of dietary improvement for adults with major depression (the "smiles" trial)'. *BMC Medicine*, vol. 15, no. 23, 30 January 2017.

44 Wiertsema, S. P. *et al.* 'The interplay between the gut microbiome and the immune system in the context of infectious diseases throughout life and the role of Nutrition in Optimizing Treatment Strategies'. *Nutrients*, vol. 13, no. 3, 9 March 2021, p. 886.

45 'Big Data from world's largest citizen science microbiome project serves food for thought'. sciencedaily.com, 15 May 2018.

46 'Eating more fruit and vegetables linked to less stress, study finds'. sciencedaily.com, 14 May 2021.

47 'Fruit and veggies give you the feel-good factor'. sciencedaily.com, 10 June 2016.

48 'The right '5-a-day' mix is 2 fruit and 3 vegetable servings for longer life'. sciencedaily.com, 1 March 2021.

49 NHS. '5-a-day: What Counts?'. nhs.uk.

50 Marles, R. J. 'Mineral nutrient composition of vegetables, fruits and grains: The context of reports of apparent historical declines'. *Journal of Food Composition and Analysis*, vol. 56, March 2017, pp. 93–103.

51 My Food Data. myfooddata.com.

52 NHS. 'Diagnosis: Obesity'. nhs.uk.

53 National Institute for Health and Care Excellence (NICE). 'Keep the size of your waist to less than half of your height, updated NICE draft guideline recommends'. nice.org.uk, 8 April 2022.

References

54 King's College London. 'New research reveals why some of us are hungry all the time'. kcl.ac.uk, 12 April 2021.

55 McArthur, B. M. *et al.* 'Mastication of nuts under realistic eating conditions: Implications for energy balance'. *Nutrients*, vol. 10, no. 6, 1 June 2018.

56 Nguyen, H. ;Consumption of several types of soft drinks remained stable year-over-year in Great Britain'. yougov.co.uk, 18 February 2021.

57 PureGym. 'Soft drinks litres per person'. puregym.com

58 'New poll charts UK coffee shop consumer attitude'. World Coffee Portal. 18 October 2021.

59 Alcohol Change UK. 'Alcohol statistics'. alcoholchange.org.uk

60 Queen Mary University of London. 'New study shows light-to-moderate coffee consumption is associated with health-benefits'. 10 February 2022, qmul.ac.uk

61 The Nutrition Source. 'Drinks to consume in moderation'. hsph.harvard.edu

62 'Large study challenges the theory that light alcohol consumption benefits heart health'. sciencedaily.com, 25 March 2022.

63 Hayward, E. 'Heavy drinkers "healthier and happier in later years"'. *The Times*, 2 June 2022.

Recipe Index

Recipe Index

Recipe Index

General Index

General Index

General Index

poultry
  cooking methods 88
  nutrition 39
prebiotics 56, 71
pregnancy 19, 29
probiotics
  foods 71 *see also*
    fermented foods
  supplements 68
processed foods
  gut microbiome 65
  trans fats 44–5
  ultra-processed foods
    (UPFs) 3, 30, 36, 66
protein
  age related requirements
    8, 14
  definition and function in
    the body 34–5
  exercise 35
  meat 35–6
  powders 37, 42
  satiety 95
  sources 36, 37, 38–40, 41–3
  summary information 41
  UK guidelines 35, 38
  weight management 34
psyllium husks 61

quinoa 29, 37, 40

rainbow trout 50, 53
raisins 94
rapeseed oil 115
recipes nutrition 112–13
Reference Nutrient Intake
  (RNI) 83
resistant starch 55–6, 61, 71
rice 29, 30, 40, 56, 59, 71
root vegetables 30, 33
Rossi, Megan 65
rye 66

salad dressings 53, 94
salads 80
salmon 50, 94
salt 81, 113, 115
sarcopenia 14
sardines 50, 53
satiety 34, 49, 95–6
saturated fats 44, 45
sauerkraut 71

seafood 42–3
seeds
  gut microbiome 71
  'hero' ingredient 114
  increasing intake 32
  nutrition 30, 40, 51
  plants, 30 different 65
  portion sizes 94
selenium 18, 85
shopping tips 32, 71, 72, 86,
  114
sleep 105
smoothies
  fibre 32
  home made 75, 106
  portion sizes 257
  protein powders 42
snacks
  blood sugar and lifestyle
    factors 97–8
  evenings 96, 101
  gut microbiome 72
  healthy options 80, 99–101
  processed foods 30
  summary information 100
  triggers and assessment 98
soluble fibre 55
soy foods
  increasing intake 43, 70–1
  nutrition 13, 37, 40, 54
Spector, Tim 6, 65
spices 65, 71, 115
spinach 32, 72
sprouts 55
starch
  definition 24
  resistant starch 55–6, 61, 71
stevia 26
stock cubes 114
stomach 15
stress 13, 73, 105
sugar 24–5, 31
sugar substitutes 25–6
supplements 16–19, 47–8, 68,
  82
sweet potatoes 30, 87

tahini 94
teenagers 8–10
tempeh 40, 43, 70–1
tofu 40

tomatoes 57, 87
trans fats 44–5
tubers 30, 33
turkey 39

ultra-processed foods (UPFs)
  3, 30, 36, 66

vagus nerve 64
vegan/vegetarian diets
  fibre 57
  micronutrients 88–9
  omega-3 48
  protein 34–5, 37
  supplements 18–19
vegetables
  box schemes 71
  complex carbohydates 32
  cooking methods 87, 88
  cruciferous 13, 55
  'eat the rainbow' 76–8
  five-a-day summary 79
  frozen 42, 72, 89
  fruit 89
  increasing intake 32, 79–80
  mental health 73
  nutrition 29, 55
  plants, 30 different 65
  portion sizes 74–5
  sugars 25
vitamin A
  food pairing 87
  sources 84, 89
  supplements and cancer
    risk 18
  UK guidelines 48
vitamin Bs 18, 84, 89
vitamin C
  age related requirements
    10
  cooking methods 88
  excess 18
  sources 10, 30, 84
  UK guidelines 83
vitamin D
  age related requirements
    9, 15
  food pairing 87, 88
  sources 9, 81, 84
  supplements 19
vitamin E 84, 87, 99
vitamin K 85, 87